Pregnancy exercise

Judy DiFiore

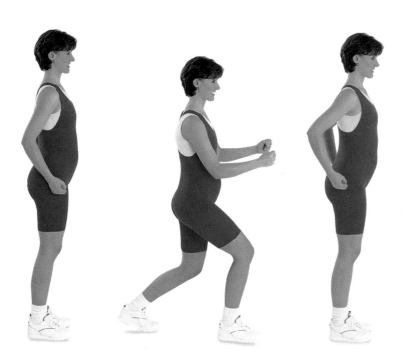

CARROLL & BROWN PUBLISHERS LIMITED

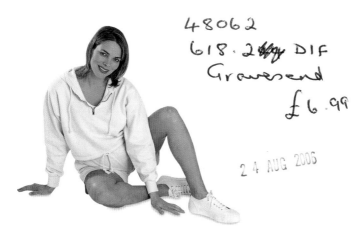

To my mum, and all the expectant mums I have worked with

This edition first published in 2006 in the United Kingdom by

CARROLL & BROWN LIMITED
20 Lonsdale Road, London NW6 6RD

Editor: Caroline Uzielli
Art Editor: Evie Loizides
Photography: Jules Selmes

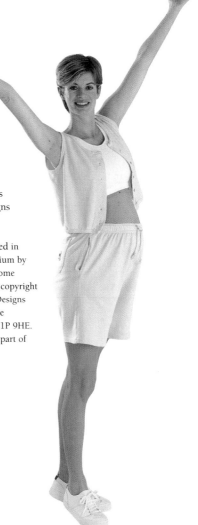

Text © 2006 Judy DiFiore
Illustrations and compilation © 2006
Carroll & Brown Limited, London

A CIP catalogue record for this book is available
from the British Library

ISBN 1-904760-41-4
ISBN-13 978-1-904760-41-2

The moral right of Judy DiFiore to be identified as author of this
work has been asserted in accordance with the Copyright, Designs
and Patents Act of 1988

Reproduced by Rali, Spain
Printed and bound in Spain by Bookprint

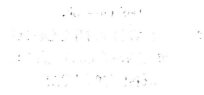

CONTENTS

FOREWORD

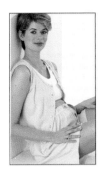

Welcome to my pregnancy exercise programme. I've designed it to help you to keep fit, increase your confidence in your changing shape and leave you feeling full of zest and vitality!

You may be wondering if it is safe to continue with your regular exercise programme or begin exercising now that you're pregnant. This book will answer your questions and help you to exercise confidently and safely until the birth. As a specialist teacher of pregnancy exercises, with years of practical experience of teaching both the fit and not-so-fit, I have a deep understanding of the changes and discomforts associated with pregnancy, and a strong awareness of how a pregnant woman feels. My programme is comprehensive yet flexible; full of modifications to make the exercises easier or harder, depending on how you feel.

Exercising regularly using this book will help you enjoy a comfortable pregnancy. It can improve your posture, relieve stiffness, aches and pains, strengthen your muscles and increase energy levels. The exercises help to control excess weight gain (if combined with sensible eating) and may encourage you to relax and sleep better. What's more, your circulation will improve, reducing discomforts such as varicose veins, leg cramps and constipation. Most importantly, your increased strength and stamina will enable you to cope better during labour.

Although you may not yet have considered what life will be like after your baby is born, your body will recover more quickly if you exercise during pregnancy. You should have more energy to cope with your new baby and increased strength for the enormous amounts of lifting and carrying involved in everyday babycare. Your abdominal and pelvic floor muscles should regain their strength sooner and you will find it easier to return to your pre-pregnancy shape and posture if your muscles remain toned and stretched.

So, what are you waiting for? Help yourself to make your pregnancy a wonderful experience. Get moving, feel confident about your beautiful body and, above all, enjoy your pregnancy.

Judy DiFiore

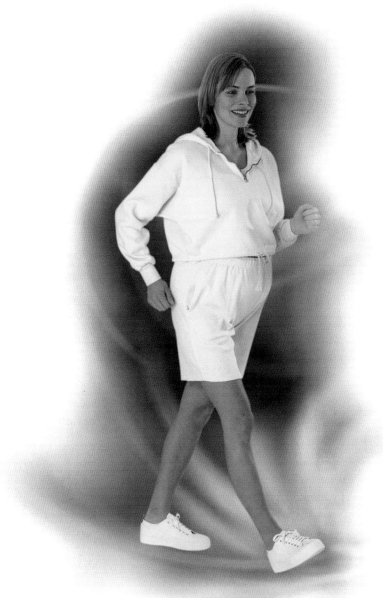

THE PREGNANCY PROGRAMME

This chapter tells you all you need to know about the exercise programme before you begin. It starts by explaining how to work out effectively and how to structure your exercise session to suit your needs. I have included five mini programmes, which take from as little as 10 minutes, to fit into the tightest of schedules. The changes that occur to your body during pregnancy and how these affect the way you exercise are discussed in detail. The final part of the chapter provides guidelines for safe exercise, highlights when exercise should be continued with caution or stop altogether and gets you suitably kitted out and ready for action.

About the workout

My special pregnancy exercise programme consists of four sections: the warm-up, which prepares your body for exercise; the aerobics section, which helps you to build stamina; the strengthening and toning exercises, which increase muscle fitness; and the stretching and relaxing section, which helps to reduce stiffness. Together they create a comprehensive workout which will leave you feeling refreshed and invigorated.

WORKING OUT EFFECTIVELY

To improve physical fitness you must exercise at a level which places greater demands on your body than your normal daily activities. By altering the frequency, intensity, time and type of exercise, your body learns to adapt to the new level of exertion and your fitness can be improved, or at least maintained if you were previously fit.

The *frequency* of your workout is important – aim to complete this programme at least three times per week, but do not exceed five sessions weekly. Try to leave one day between workouts to allow your body time to rest and recover.

It is also important to monitor the *intensity* of your workout to ensure that it is sufficiently demanding to be beneficial.

A total workout *time* of one hour is recommended, but do not exceed 90 minutes. Avoid increasing the time and intensity simultaneously; either keep the intensity as before and continue for longer, or increase the level but work out for the same time.

This *type* of exercise programme provides a comprehensive workout to improve and/or maintain cardiovascular and muscular fitness. However, other suitable exercises include swimming or aqua-natal classes, brisk walking and cycling.

How hard should you work? This depends on the amount of exercise you took previously, the stage of your pregnancy and how energetic you are feeling on the day you work out.

The exercises in this programme have been devised to accommodate all these factors, and include guidelines for three different activity levels: "gentle," "moderate" and "energetic". The technique for each exercise is unaffected by the activity level; the "moderate" and "energetic" levels simply require that you work at a higher intensity or for longer than the "gentle" level. If you turn to the step-by-step exercise sequences, you will see that each page features three circular, orange symbols; these detail instructions for each activity level. You can follow any of the levels during pregnancy, but guidelines are as follows:

GENTLE — *Follow this level if you took no exercise before pregnancy, you are returning to exercise after a break or you are feeling particularly tired.*

MODERATE — *This level is suitable if you exercised occasionally before pregnancy or if you have always enjoyed a fairly active lifestyle.*

ENERGETIC — *This is an ideal level if you exercised two or three times per week before pregnancy and continue to do so now or if you are feeling full of vitality.*

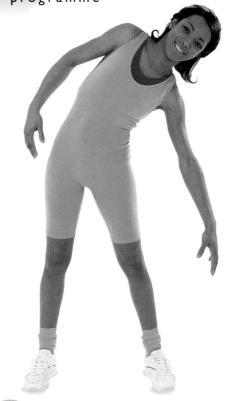

WARMING UP

It is essential to prepare your body for any physical activity by warming up as this will help to prevent injury and make the exercises feel more comfortable.

The warm-up section consists of two types of exercise. The first 11 exercises are mobility exercises, which warm and loosen your body and make your muscles more pliable and less likely to pull. The last eight are stretching exercises, which help to relieve muscular tension caused by the postural changes of pregnancy and lengthen your muscles in a controlled way before you use them more vigorously in the following two sections of the programme. There is no differentiation between the three levels – "relaxed," "moderate" and "energetic" – all the exercises should be performed the same, regardless of your fitness level.

How long should it take? This section can be completed in 10 minutes. You must perform all the warm-up exercises before doing the aerobics section.

WORKING THROUGH THIS SECTION

▶ First, you must remember to free up your joints – shoulders, spine, hips, knees and ankles – by taking them through their natural range of movement; start with small moves and then gradually increase the size. Move each joint several times and feel it loosening and getting warmer as your movements increase.

▶ The mobilizing exercises can be done in any order, but the stretches must be performed at the end of the warm-up when you feel warmer and looser.

▶ Next, boost your circulation and warm up your muscles by making large, controlled leg movements which also incorporate a small amount of arm work, such as knee raises, knee bends and marching in place. You will become warmer fairly quickly so this part of the warm-up need not be too long.

▶ Lastly, stretch all the muscles you intend to work later; if you are planning an upper body workout, for example, do all the upper body stretches. Also, you should stretch any muscles that are feeling stiff now that you're pregnant, such as those at the front of the hips and the chest.

▶ Alternatively, you can easily warm up by going for a fairly brisk five minute walk. When you return home, you can then perform all the mobility exercises, as well as the stretches.

AEROBIC EXERCISE

This is any type of low-level physical activity – such as walking, swimming or cycling – which, continued for a period of time, increases your heart rate, makes you a little out of breath, builds up your strength and stamina, and gives your body an even workout. To gain any physical benefit, exercise should be continuous for at least 20 minutes (30 minutes at the most), and the amount of effort you put into the exercises should be high enough to make you feel slightly out of breath.

The exercises in this section are designed to be repeated, but the amount of repetitions vary according to your level of fitness and stage of pregnancy (*see page vi*). Repeat all the exercises you do in this section in reverse order to ensure that you receive a full workout and to give your body a chance to cool down.

THE BORG SCALE

RPE SCALE	INTENSITY
6, 7, 8	extremely light
9, 10	light
11, 12	fairly light
13, 14	*moderately hard*
15, 16	hard
17, 18	very hard
19, 20	extremely hard

Assessing aerobic intensity Each exercise in this section can be performed at three different levels: "gentle", "moderate" or "energetic" (*see page vi*). The amount of effort you put into your aerobic exercise, however, must be monitored carefully to ensure that you are gaining fitness benefits, but are not overexerting yourself. To do this use the Borg scale (*see above*) and/or the talk test.

The Borg scale, devised by the Swedish psychophysiologist Gunnar Borg, is based on your subjective rate of perceived exertion (RPE). It requires you to assess how hard you *feel* you are working on a scale of 6–20. The recommended intensity for pregnancy is between 13–14 which is "moderately hard" on the Borg scale. If the exercise feels exhausting, slow down: follow the "gentle" instructions if you have been exercising at the "moderate" or "energetic" levels.

The talk test works as follows. You should be able to hold a conversation while exercising at the recommended level without gasping for air. If your breathing is heavy and laboured you are working too hard; you *should* feel a little out of breath, however, otherwise you are unlikely to see any long-term fitness benefits.

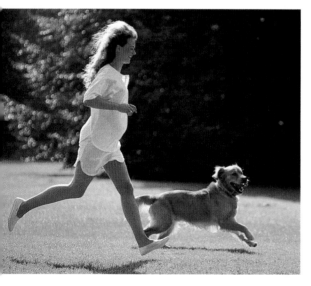

Exercise for fun
Make exercise enjoyable and part of your daily routine. Outdoor aerobic activity, such as light jogging or brisk walking, can help to lift your spirits and give your body an overall workout.

WORKING THROUGH THIS SECTION

▶ Begin by repeating each exercise a few times to familiarize yourself with the rhythm, coordination and technique required; but do not tire your muscles. Then, work through the exercises, repeating each one according to your chosen level. If you are lacking in energy, do not feel that you *must* perform all the exercises; just select a few.

▶ Always start with low-level movements and gradually increase the intensity by using larger movements or increasing the involvement of the arms; this will give your body time to meet the demands for more oxygen, making the exercises much more comfortable to do, and will enable you to continue for longer.

▶ If you are feeling especially tired or have little energy, take short breaks between the exercises by marching in place.

▶ Reduce the arm work if it becomes too demanding and rest your hands on your hips for a short while. Add the arms back into the movement when you feel ready.

▶ Keep your movements at a steady, controlled pace throughout and take particular care of your pelvis as the movements become larger.

▶ The intensity of your exercises should decrease in exactly the same way as they increased, so having completed the desired number of exercises, you must then repeat them all in reverse order, giving your heart rate time to slow and your body a chance to cool down a little.

▶ When you feel ready, increase your workout by adding one or two more exercises but remember that you must

CAUTION

• Always exercise at a gentle/moderate level (*see Borg Scale and talk test on page viii*). Do not overexert yourself; pregnancy is not a time to achieve your fitness goals.
• Avoid overheating. If you live in a hot climate, exercise during cool times of the day, such as early morning or evening, or use a fan in your exercise area.
• Be sure to exercise in a well-ventilated room; and avoid dehydration by taking regular sips of water.
• Exercise should never suddenly stop. Aerobic exercise causes an increase in your heart rate and promotes blood flow to your working muscles; standing still for long periods may cause you to feel faint or dizzy as your circulation struggles to return the blood to your heart.
• Avoid performing the aerobic exercises on their own; you must always do the warm-up beforehand and stretch out afterwards.
• Avoid rapid changes of direction which may cause damage to your joints.

repeat them all in reverse order before stopping.

▶ Gradually build up to include all the exercises. When you become more familiar with the movements you can mix and match them into a variety of combinations, or if you are feeling especially active, you can follow the instructions in the "Feeling Energetic" boxes. Always ensure that you allow yourself sufficient recovery time.

How long should it take? Try to exercise continuously for 20 minutes, although if you are fairly new to exercise, 10 minutes will probably be sufficient. If you feel like it, you can continue for longer, but you should avoid exceeding 30 minutes.

STRENGTHENING AND TONING

This section consists of exercises for individual muscle groups. By performing several continuous repetitions of the same exercise, you place extra demands on the muscle which then adapts and becomes stronger. Strength and tone can be increased further by working the muscles against a resistance, such as your body weight or gravity. Remember to perform each exercise several times (known as repetitions or reps); groups of reps are known as sets. The recommended number of reps are given for each exercise and vary according to the exercise, position used, the three levels of fitness and your stage of pregnancy.

How long should it take? This will depend upon how many exercises you select. Aim to do at least 20 minutes and always perform the abdominal and pelvic floor exercises.

WORKING THROUGH THIS SECTION

▶ Start this section with three or four exercises to familiarize yourself with the technique. Select the areas you want to work but keep a balance of upper and lower body work, and combine these with the essential abdominal and pelvic floor exercises. It is important to ensure that you take a short break between each set of reps to give your muscles time to rest and recover before being challenged again.

CAUTION

- Due to the changes that take place to your abdominals during pregnancy, the abdominal exercises in this programme have been divided into those appropriate for the first trimester, and those appropriate for the second and third trimesters.
- Some exercises may feel uncomfortable or make you become a little light-headed or dizzy, especially during your third trimester. If this is the case, follow the seated versions of the standing toning exercises.

▶ Your muscles should begin to ache after a few repetitions, but try not to give up immediately (unless it is very painful). The standing leg exercises often cause your supporting leg to tire before the working leg, so it may be necessary to stop and shake out both legs before continuing. Remember to check your body positioning before restarting.

▶ Some muscles need to be worked with light weights or resistance bands (cans of food will do!) in order to be worked effectively. All the exercises in this section should be performed *slowly* and with control, not only for the safety of your muscles and joints but also to ensure maximum physical benefit.

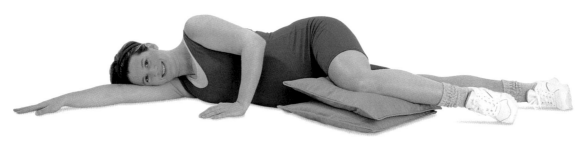

STRETCHING AND RELAXING

This is the final part of your workout. It gives your body a chance to recover from the more vigorous activities of the previous sections and provides an opportunity to relax.

During exercise your muscles have to contract, and if the movements are repeated your muscles may remain in a slightly shortened state. Stretching at the end of your workout when your muscles are really warm will help to keep you supple and mobile and will also extend your muscles back to their original length. You must stretch slowly and with control when pregnant to avoid overextending your joints or pulling your muscles. As with the warm-up, there is no differentiation between the three levels; all the exercises should be performed the same.

Finding the time to relax This can become increasingly difficult as we try to squeeze more into our busy lives. A short period of relaxation at the end of your workout, or whenever possible, will help to reduce any muscular tension and will also leave you feeling refreshed and invigorated. Regular relaxation sessions can also help you to feel more in tune with your body and may even help you to relax during labour and after the birth.

How long should it take? In order to be thorough and effective, this section should not be rushed. The stretches will take at least 5 minutes to complete and time spent on the relaxation and wake-up can vary between 5 and 15 minutes.

WORKING THROUGH THIS SECTION

▶ Only stretch when your muscles are warm as they are softer, more pliable and less likely to injure. If alternative positions are given, choose the most comfortable.

▶ Try to hold all the stretching positions for 6–8 seconds; some of the more comfortable positions, however, could be held for longer. Where appropriate, make sure you relax the rest of your body.

▶ Move slowly and with control into each stretch until you experience a feeling of mild tension in the relevant muscle. If the stretch becomes painful, you must stop immediately.

▶ After the stretching exercises, you should allow time to rest and relax. A selection of positions are provided in this programme so you can choose the most comfortable or appropriate. Remain in the position for as long as you can; you may be surprised at how refreshed you feel after just a few minutes of relaxation.

▶ Always allow sufficient time to fully wake up and recover after you have finished this section. Avoid standing up suddenly after relaxing as you could become dizzy or light-headed.

FINDING THE TIME TO EXERCISE

Fitting exercise into your busy lifestyle may be the most difficult part of this programme, but it is important to remain committed to exercise in order to reap the benefits. I have devised several mini programmes that take less than 35 minutes to complete (*see page xiii*) in order to encourage you to find time to work out. If these programmes are impractical for daily participation there are other ways you can include exercise in your routine.

Opportunities to exercise Regular repetition of the postural and loosening exercises (*see pages 2–11*) throughout the day can have a significant effect on your body and you will be surprised at just how much can be achieved in relatively little time.

Posture checks, pelvic floors and abdominal exercises can be done anywhere and as often as possible during the day, and you can even exercise when seated (*see below*). If you need a reminder, put some coloured stickers in prominent places around your home or office, such as in the bathroom, on the refrigerator door, with your car keys or even on the office fax machine to make sure that you never miss an opportunity to exercise. Your colleagues and friends will be intrigued and may want to join in too!

▶ Take the stairs rather than using the lift; you can always have a breather on the way up if you need to.

▶ Go for a walk during your lunch break. If possible, leave your coat and heavy bags behind and enjoy the freedom of your arms swinging gently as you increase the pace.

▶ Go for a swim or join an aqua-natal class; your body will feel great supported by the water which, if used correctly, can help to provide a very effective full body workout.

▶ Before getting into the bath or when lying in bed, tighten your abdominals and watch your baby being lifted up into you.

seated exercises

Neck and shoulders Circle your shoulders slowly back and around, then tip your head gently over to each side. Pause briefly each side.

Chest and spine Slowly squeeze your shoulder blades together to open your chest, and release. Reach your arm down to one side and bend your upper body slowly over; then repeat on the other side. Reach each arm up to the ceiling and hold for a few seconds; repeat.

Lower back and abdominal muscles Sitting on a sturdy, upright chair tilt your pelvis, curl your back and press your lower back into the chair. Then, tighten your abdominal muscles and lift your baby up and in towards you.

Feet and ankles With one foot off the floor, slowly and gently circle the ankle until it feels looser; repeat with the other foot. Then, lift and lower your heels several times keeping your toes on the floor.

Pelvic floor exercises Tighten your pelvic floor muscles using both the fast and slow speeds (*see page 43*).

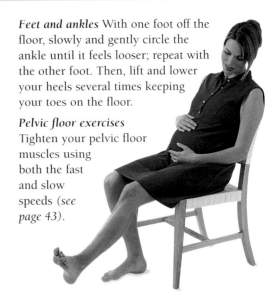

MINI PROGRAMMES

I have designed the following mini exercise programmes to give you some ideas of how to structure your workout to meet your needs and fit it into your schedule. You could create your own programme by mixing and matching other exercises in this book; the purpose of each exercise is given at the top of every page so you can select those most appropriate for your chosen workout. Try to avoid repeating the same plan – if you choose the upper body plan one day, perform the lower body plan on the next occasion. By varying your workouts, you will keep yourself motivated and gain maximum fitness benefits.

10 MINS
REVITALIZING PLAN

WARMING UP
All exercises.

STRETCHING & RELAXING
All seated stretches.

15 MINS
GENTLE PLAN

WARMING UP
All exercises.

STRENGTHENING & TONING
Pelvic floors, head and shoulder raise and kneeling abdominal curl.

20 MINS
UPPER BODY PLAN

WARMING UP
All warming and loosening exercises.
Stretches for side muscles, triceps and pectorals.

STRENGTHENING & TONING
Biceps curl, pelvic floors, abdominal curl, press up, shoulder shrug and shoulder squeeze; perform all these exercises, then repeat.

STRETCHING & RELAXING
Seated stretches for pectorals, triceps and side muscles.

30 MINS
LOWER BODY PLAN

WARMING UP
All warming and loosening exercises.
Stretches for calf muscles, quadriceps, hip flexors and adductors.

STRENGTHENING & TONING
Forward lunge, calf raise, pelvic floors, abdominal curls, outer thigh raise and inner thigh raise.

STRETCHING & RELAXING
Seated stretches for hamstrings, adductors and gluteals.
Standing stretches for quadriceps, calf muscles and hip flexors.

35 MINS
CARDIO PLAN

WARMING UP
All warming and loosening exercises.
Stretches for calf muscles, quadriceps, hip flexors and adductors.

AEROBICS
Selection of movements from the range
OR 20-minute brisk walk.

STRETCHING & RELAXING
Seated stretches for hamstrings, adductors and gluteals.
Standing stretches for quadriceps, calf muscles and hip flexors.

Understanding your changing body

Apart from the very obvious changes to your shape during pregnancy, your body undergoes other changes, many of which you should be aware of when exercising.

RAISED HORMONE LEVELS

Your body experiences numerous hormonal changes, some of which influence the way you exercise; three hormones are most relevant to exercise – relaxin, oestrogen and progesterone.

Effects on exercise It is important to take account of these hormonal changes when you work out. Exercises that were previously unproblematic may become inappropriate now that you're pregnant.

▶ When your body weight is forward and supported on your hands and knees (kneeling on all fours), you may experience a tingling sensation or a numbness in your fingers; this is due to water retention. You may also get heartburn when in this position, which is due to the effects of progesterone on your digestive system.

▶ Your ankles may become swollen, which will make it uncomfortable to wear trainers for any length of time. This footwear is recommended for the aerobic section, but can be removed for other sections. Swollen ankles may be due to water retention, but they can also indicate raised

blood pressure, so you should check this before continuing.

▶ Reduced joint stability, due to relaxin, may increase the risk of injury. Your pelvis and spine are particularly vulnerable due to the forward pull of your baby and decreased support from your stretched abdominals, so correct posture and good exercise technique are vital. Avoid high-impact or bouncy movements as they increase the stress to your joints, breasts and pelvic floor.

▶ You will feel warmer quickly because your body temperature is already raised due to progesterone. You should avoid getting too hot and must always exercise in a well-ventilated room.

▶ During the aerobic section, keep your legs moving to assist the return of blood back to the heart. If you stop suddenly you may feel dizzy due to the influence of progesterone dilating the walls of your blood vessels.

Relaxin softens the connective tissue in joints and muscles enabling the pelvis to widen for delivery and the abdominals and pelvic floor muscles to stretch.

Oestrogen is the growth hormone. It causes your breasts to enlarge and increases the size and strength of your heart. It also encourages water retention.

Progesterone relaxes the walls of the blood vessels, to enable them to cope with the increased volume of blood. It also increases your body temperature.

YOUR ABDOMINAL MUSCLES

These muscles support your growing uterus and will help you to push your baby out during the second stage of labour. They also keep your abdomen pulled in, allow you to move your trunk in a variety of directions, support the lower back and abdominal organs, and brace your body when you are lifting.

WHERE TO LOCATE THEM

The layers of your abdominal muscles form an abdominal wall – a very strong, natural girdle around your middle. They extend vertically from your ribs and breastbone down to the top of your pelvis, and diagonally and horizontally from your sides inward.

Making room for your baby During pregnancy your abdominal muscles undergo a huge amount of stretching in all directions under the influence of the hormone relaxin. Your waistline can increase from approximately 66 cm (26 inches) to 117 cm (46 inches) and the muscles may lengthen vertically from 30 cm (12 inches) to 51 cm (20 inches). In order for this degree of growth to occur, the abdominal muscles have to stretch away from their central position. This opening out of the muscle bands gives your baby room to grow; it is not painful and you may even be unaware it has occurred.

Abdominal exercise Simple abdominal exercises should be part of your daily routine, and because the exercises can be performed almost anywhere, they can be performed repeatedly throughout the day. Strong abdominals will help you to maintain a degree of tone in your abdomen and reduce backache by taking the strain of the frontal load away from your back. If you have not exercised these muscles before, then you need to start immediately – they do still work during pregnancy and will respond well if exercised. If you previously performed curl-up strengthening exercises for the abdominals, it is *not* recommended that you continue to do so once the muscles have begun to stretch; they may separate and weaken further. By the time you reach 16 weeks, however, you should follow the second and third trimester abdominal exercises (*see pages 47–49*), although you may need to change sooner if you are not comfortable lying on your back. If these exercises make your muscles ache, release them for a moment and try again. The more you practise, the stronger the muscles will become and the longer you will be able to hold the positions.

Easy, everyday abdominal exercises
These will strengthen those muscles that protect your baby and your back. Pull your clothes firmly across the abdomen, tighten your abdominals and watch as your baby lifts up and in towards you; if your muscles are strong the degree of movement will amaze you.

YOUR PELVIC FLOOR MUSCLES

Under the influence of relaxin and the increasing weight of your growing baby, your pelvic floor muscles weaken and begin to stretch. This may cause the sphincters (rings of muscle, *see box below*) to widen and become less effective at resisting internal pressure, resulting in a small leak of urine when you cough, sneeze, or laugh. This condition, known as stress incontinence, is not uncommon during pregnancy but tends to be most prevalent in the early postnatal period due to the stretching and weakening that takes place during labour and delivery. Daily pelvic floor exercises, sometimes known as Kegels, may help to prevent or alleviate this problem.

Prevention is better than cure Strong pelvic floor muscles will help during delivery and aid the healing process following the birth. Exercises for the pelvic floor muscles should commence as soon as you know that you are pregnant. It is better to strengthen these muscles before the weight of the baby begins to exert increased pressure, rather than trying to locate and work them when they are already stretched and weakened. Slow and fast pelvic floor exercises are featured on *page 43*. Practise both on a daily basis: the slow ones will help you to develop the strength needed to support your baby in the third trimester, while the fast ones will help to prevent stress incontinence.

Regular repetition
Try to associate pelvic floor exercises with a regular daily activity – every time you answer the telephone, for example – so that you perform them several times throughout the day.

Working your pelvic floor muscles Try these exercises in a seated position initially; you should find it easier when your body weight is supported. If you cannot feel anything happening, next time you go to the toilet try stopping the flow of urine midstream (preferably not with a full bladder). The strength of the pelvic floor muscles is determined by their ability to stop the flow of urine. Be sure to release your muscles and allow the bladder to empty afterwards. This procedure should be used only as a method of locating these muscles, *not* as your daily exercise, as it carries an increased risk of infection. Initially you will probably need to stop what you are doing and concentrate hard when trying to exercise your pelvic floor muscles, but don't worry, it will feel much easier and more natural as you become more experienced; don't give up after the first few attempts.

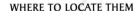

WHERE TO LOCATE THEM

The pelvic floors form a hammock between the front and back of your pelvis and support your pelvic and abdominal organs: the bladder, uterus, and the bowel. Additional "rings" of muscle, called sphincters, encircle the urethra and vagina at the front, and the anus at the back.

PERFECTING PREGNANCY POSTURE

Correct posture is essential for reducing the physical stress to your body during pregnancy. Before you begin any workout, it is important to run through the key points for correct posture (*see page 2*) – they are easy to achieve and should be practised at every opportunity throughout the day.

Postural changes in pregnancy At the beginning of your pregnancy your uterus is tucked away in your pelvis, but as your pregnancy progresses, it slowly rises up into the abdomen. It is at this stage that your posture begins to dramatically change. The weight of your baby will tip your pelvis forward and, as your baby continues to grow, your abdominal muscles will stretch. You will have a natural tendency to compensate for this increased frontal load by leaning slightly back; but this can put pressure on your lower spine and may cause considerable pain and discomfort in your back.

The increased weight of your breasts may pull on your upper back and cause you to stand with rounded shoulders and sunken chest. This may cause excess strain on your upper back and restrict the space in your ribcage, making breathing more difficult.

Exercises to protect your back A strong back is essential during pregnancy so your body can cope with the increased frontal load. Strengthening and stretching certain muscles will protect your back against any long-term problems and will help you to maintain a good posture throughout your pregnancy.

▶ Strengthening your abdominal muscles (*see pages 44–49*) will help to reduce lower backache as these muscles take the strain of the extra frontal load away from your back.

▶ Stretching your hip flexors (*see pages 17 and 72*) will enable you to correctly tilt your pelvis and prevent your back from arching; if these muscles are tight, it will be difficult to do this correctly. Strengthening your buttock muscles (*see pages 37 and 54*) and abdominals (*see pages 44–49*) will help you to maintain this position.

▶ Stretching and lengthening your pectorals (*see pages 19 and 61*) will help you to open your chest. Strengthening your upper back muscles (*see pages 51–52*) will keep your shoulders back and reduce upper back strain.

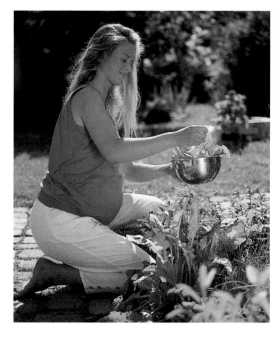

Maintaining perfect posture
Back care is vital for all activities during pregnancy. When bending down, keep your pelvis tilted and abdominals tight; bend from your knees and use your leg muscles to kneel down and stand up.

Working out sensibly

Whatever your stage of pregnancy, exercise will be beneficial as it can reduce many common discomforts, ease postnatal recovery and, not least, promote a sense of well-being. It is important to be cautious, however – listen to your body, be aware of your changing capabilities, and ensure that you always follow the exercise guidelines and safety concerns detailed on *pages xx–xxi*.

THE THREE TRIMESTERS

Pregnancy is divided into three phases of roughly 13 weeks each, known as trimesters. During each trimester you will experience a variety of physiological changes and symptoms, and you will need to re-evaluate your exercise routine to take account of them. It is important to remember that pregnancy is *not* a time to recondition your body or set fitness targets. You should be looking to maintain, or slightly improve (if previously unfit), your strength and stamina.

You can continue this exercise programme during all three trimesters, but you must always listen to your body. If you're fit and full of get-up-and-go, you can follow the "energetic" level of activity well into your third trimester (*see page vi*). When you're feeling particularly tired, however, adjust the intensity of your workout to the "gentle" level. Don't worry if you find that you're changing your activity level from one day to the next, or from one stage of pregnancy to the next – this is perfectly natural, and a good sign that you're sensitive to your own needs.

YOUR FIRST TRIMESTER: WEEKS 1–13

As soon as your egg is fertilized your body begins the amazing process to motherhood. During the next few weeks, however, pregnancy symptoms may not make you feel like rushing out and celebrating.

IS IT SAFE TO EXERCISE?

If your pregnancy is progressing normally and you are used to physical activity, the answer is yes. If you are a newcomer to exercise, you should begin this programme very gradually and with care. It may be the last thing you feel like doing, however, so don't force yourself.

EXERCISE GUIDELINES

This is the most fragile stage of pregnancy and crucial to the formation of the fetus, so observe the following points:
• Don't get too hot; excess heat is passed on to the baby. Avoid saunas and sunbeds until after your baby is born.
• Always exercise in a well-ventilated room.
• Take regular sips of water to prevent dehydration.

EXERCISE BENEFITS

Gentle exercise can help to reduce unpleasant symptoms caused by surging hormone levels. Sickness or nausea can occur at any time of the day and exercise may help to reduce these feelings. Exercise is a good pick-me-up and can help to boost energy levels, but if you are totally exhausted, rest whenever possible. To reduce pain and tenderness in the breasts wear a good supporting bra.

YOUR SECOND TRIMESTER: WEEKS 14–26

You are now entering a great stage of pregnancy when you will probably feel better than ever. Sickness and nausea usually cease and your energy will return.

IS IT SAFE TO EXERCISE?

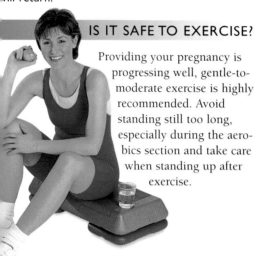

Providing your pregnancy is progressing well, gentle-to-moderate exercise is highly recommended. Avoid standing still too long, especially during the aerobics section and take care when standing up after exercise.

EXERCISE GUIDELINES

Your pregnancy may now begin to show, so back care is a main priority.
• Avoid any high-impact activities or bouncy movements.
• Don't exercise on your back as the baby's weight can restrict blood flow back to your heart. Follow the second trimester exercises.
• Allow plenty of time when changing positions during the floorwork.

EXERCISE BENEFITS

As your baby grows and your body adapts to physical and hormonal changes you may experience some new complaints – but the good news is that exercise can relieve many of these symptoms. It can reduce the general aches and pains of pregnancy and keep you full of energy. The aerobic exercises in this programme (see pages 21–35) may help to relieve constipation and cramps. Ensure that you have adequate rest.

YOUR THIRD TRIMESTER: WEEKS 27–42

There are now just three months to go until your due date and the increased frontal load can cause tiredness, clumsiness and sleeping problems. But, be proud of your new shape – you'll soon be a mum!

IS IT SAFE TO EXERCISE?

If you feel up to it and have plenty of energy, then continue to exercise. If you feel tired, try performing just the warming and loosening exercises (see pages 2–11); these will help to keep you mobile and reduce muscular and joint stiffness. Avoid standing for long periods and ensure that you allow yourself sufficient time to rest and relax.

EXERCISE GUIDELINES

Your baby's size and weight will increase considerably during these last three months, making your back even more vulnerable.
• Remember to tilt your pelvis and tighten your abdominals at all times, and take care when moving from one position to another.
• Keep your movements controlled and avoid rushing the exercises; a few selected exercises performed correctly will be more beneficial.
• You may prefer to reduce your exercise intensity to a lower level. Omit any movements you find difficult.

EXERCISE BENEFITS

Gentle exercises, especially those in the relaxing section (see pages 56–73) can aid the onset of sleep, as you may have difficulty getting comfortable at night. These exercises can also help to reduce anxiety about the birth.

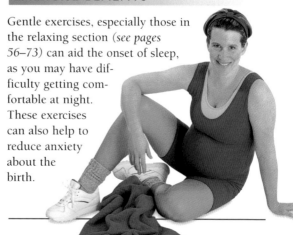

EXERCISE GUIDELINES

During pregnancy the following points should be observed to ensure that you are working out safely and not overexerting yourself or causing harm to your baby.

Don't overdo it Exercise within your limitations and avoid the temptation to push yourself. Do not exercise to exhaustion and stop when you feel fatigued – exercise should exhilarate, not drain you. Try to pitch the intensity of your workout at a level appropriate to how you are feeling (*see the Borg scale and talk test, page viii*) and remember that exercises which were easily manageable during your second trimester will probably feel much more difficult in your third trimester, so listen to your body and always err on the side of caution.

Make sure your technique is correct Follow the instructions carefully and repeat the movements slowly and with control to avoid overextending or locking out your joints, which can lead to injury. Take particular care of your back, abdominals and pelvis, especially if you are using weights.

Don't get too hot
Avoid becoming overheated, particularly in the first trimester. If you do feel yourself becoming too warm, reduce the level of your workout a little or take a short break; make sure that you have a few sips of water before continuing to exercise.

Avoid exercising on your back From 16 weeks onwards, you may begin to feel dizzy or nauseous when you lie on your back (roll on to your side immediately if you do). This programme does not include exercises which involve lying on your back from the second trimester onwards and I recommend that you avoid this position at any time after 20 weeks.

Avoid high-impact exercises Jumping movements and excessively energetic activities are not recommended after the first trimester as they increase the stress to the joints, pelvic floor muscles and breasts, and may also feel uncomfortable. Fast knee-bending movements are also unsuitable. Don't attempt any activities that require balance in the third trimester.

Breathe naturally Avoid holding your breath at any time. This may be a temptation, especially during the strengthening and toning exercises, but breath-holding can affect your blood pressure and increase the workload on your heart.

Consume extra calories An additional 300 calories per day are required to provide extra energy to cope with the pregnancy, and you need a little more than this if you are exercising regularly.

SAFETY CONCERNS

If your pregnancy is progressing well, regular exercise can be very beneficial. It is vital, however, to know when exercise can be continued with modifications and when it should stop.

When to take care Remember to listen to your body while exercising. If you experience discomfort of any sort you should check your technique or avoid that particular exercise.

▶ Avoid overheating and don't push yourself to exercise particularly during the early weeks of pregnancy.

▶ Towards the end of your pregnancy you may experience Braxton Hicks' contractions in which the abdomen tightens as the uterus contracts in practice for labour. You may wish to stop exercising while they last, but you can continue once they have subsided, providing they do not become strong and persistent.

▶ If you feel discomfort around the pubic bone, take care not to step your feet out too wide; perform the inner thigh exercises very carefully or omit them altogether.

▶ If exercising conditions are hot and humid at any time during your pregnancy, you may find it difficult to cool down after intense exercise, so choose lower-level activities.

▶ Accept the fact that on some days you may feel particularly tired and not feel like doing anything; gentle exercise can help to revitalize you, but remember to work at a level that reflects your energy and motivation at that particular time.

stop exercising immediately if...

...you experience persistent Braxton Hicks' contractions During your third trimester, it is likely that these practice contractions may become quite intense. Strong, continuous tightening must not be ignored and rest is essential.

...you feel dizzy or light-headed This could indicate low blood pressure or low blood sugar, and may be particularly noticeable if you stand still for any length of time. If you have eaten a light snack a few hours before exercise and still experience dizziness, you should have your blood pressure checked by a doctor.

...you're suffering pelvic discomfort Pain at the front or back of the pelvis may indicate increased movement of the pelvic joints. This may resolve itself with rest, but if symptoms persist you should seek immediate medical advice.

...you're exhausted Don't push yourself to exercise. If you feel overwhelming fatigue, you should relax.

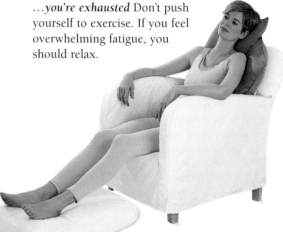

CAUTION

Seek immediate medical advice for the following:
• Abdominal or pelvic pain
• Waters breaking
• Excessive vaginal discharge
• Persistent severe headaches
• Sudden swelling of hands and ankles
• Bleeding at any stage of pregnancy (spotting a small amount of blood may occur in early pregnancy when your period would have been due).

BEFORE YOU BEGIN

Proper preparation is essential for a safe and enjoyable workout, so before you get down to exercising, make sure that you…

Wear the right gear If appropriate, you should wear several layers of clothing – this will enable you to remove garments as you become warmer. Make sure that you wear a good supporting bra, or two bras, to minimize breast movement. All the exercises, except for the aerobic section, can be performed bare-footed or in trainers; don't just wear socks as you may slip.

Keep drinking Ensure that you put some water nearby so you are able to take small sips during your workout to prevent dehydration. Have a longer drink once you're finished.

Eat before your workout So you have plenty of energy for your workout, try to eat a light meal based on complex carbohydrates such as wholewheat bread, pasta, rice, and potatoes, three or more hours before exercising. If you exercise on an empty stomach you may start to feel dizzy or light-headed; if you eat immediately before working out, however, you may suffer from heartburn. Follow your workout with a healthy snack, such as a banana or a sandwich.

Have enough space and equipment Ensure that your exercise area is free of furniture and other obstructions. You will need sufficient space to move in all directions freely and to lie down on the floor. Keep a high-backed, sturdy chair nearby or clear a stretch of wall to use as support during the standing exercises. You may need a towel or mat for the floorwork and some small hand weights – cans of food will do! A resistance band may also be handy.

Avoid interruptions Take the telephone off the hook or switch on your answerphone – this is your personal time, and once you get going, you won't want to stop.

Choose motivational music This can help you to get in the mood and make exercise more fun, but it must have a steady, moderate beat to encourage careful movement. If you exercise to music that's too fast, you risk damaging your joints and muscles. If you're not sure your music is suitable, keep the volume low; background music will increase your enjoyment and you could even sing along!

Clothing and footwear
You need to be able to move freely, so choose clothes that do not restrict your movements or dig into your abdomen. Trainers are essential for the aerobic section to support your ankles.

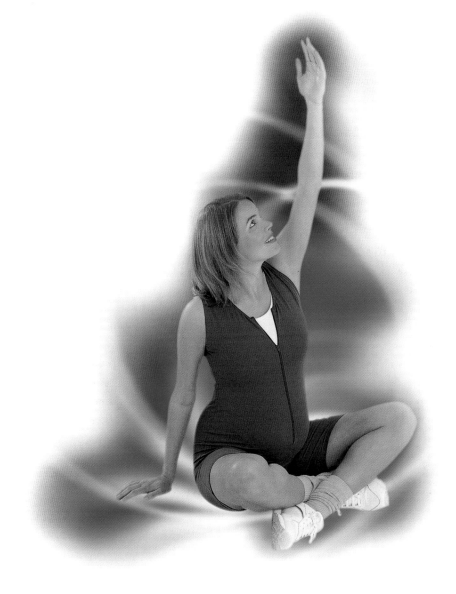

WARMING UP

These mobility exercises and stretches are essential preparation for your workout. They get your body ready for action and reduce the risk of injury, which is particularly important during pregnancy when your body is more vulnerable. After warming up, you will find the main exercise routines far easier and more comfortable to perform. What's more, the warm-up offers a perfect opportunity for you to get to know how your pregnant body feels when you move it. As you work through this section, you will be able to correct your posture and become aware of how to keep your body correctly aligned when exercising.

Posture check

To protect the back and minimize the strain on your muscles and joints

These general guidelines are important for all exercises in order to reduce the physical stress to your body during pregnancy. Practise correct posture techniques not only before you begin each exercise, but at every opportunity throughout the day.

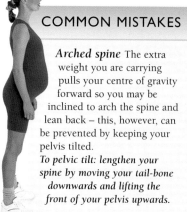

COMMON MISTAKES

Arched spine The extra weight you are carrying pulls your centre of gravity forward so you may be inclined to arch the spine and lean back – this, however, can be prevented by keeping your pelvis tilted.

To pelvic tilt: lengthen your spine by moving your tail-bone downwards and lifting the front of your pelvis upwards.

1

Stand with your feet slightly more than hip-width apart and relax your arms by your sides. Distribute your weight evenly between both feet and make sure that you keep the whole of each foot flat on the floor.

2

Lengthen your spine by lifting up out of your hips to add a couple of inches to your torso and extra space around your rib cage.

3

Tilt your pelvis (*see box, top right*) in order to keep the natural curves in your back, and tighten your abdominal muscles to lift your baby and support your lower back.

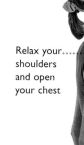

Relax your shoulders and open your chest

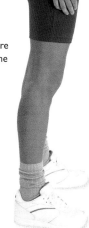

Look straight ahead and lengthen your neck, keeping your chin parallel to the floor

Tighten your abdominals

Keep your pelvis tilted

Ensure that your knees are soft and in line with your ankles

Shoulder roll

To warm and loosen your shoulders

GENTLE   MODERATE   ENERGETIC

8 reps with each shoulder

1 Stand with your feet just over hip-width apart, with your arms relaxed by your sides. Tilt the pelvis and tighten the abdominals. Rotate your right shoulder forwards; make sure you move slowly and with control.

2 Keeping the rest of your body still, raise your right shoulder up towards your ear in a steady and fluid movement; avoid tipping your head towards your raised shoulder.

3 Circle your right shoulder behind you in a large, exaggerated manner to emphasize this backwards movement. Stand tall and keep your pelvis tilted throughout.

Ensure that your feet are flat on the floor.........

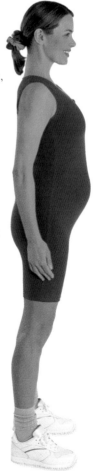

4 Take the right shoulder down, keeping your abdominals tight and your chest lifted. Remember to keep your movements slow and controlled and try to keep the knees, neck and shoulders relaxed. Continue as directed, then switch to the left shoulder.

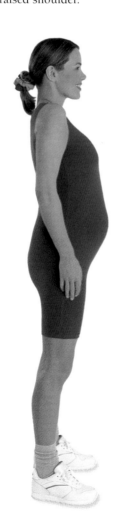

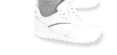

Knee bend

To warm and loosen the knees and to increase your body temperature

GENTLE   MODERATE   ENERGETIC

All levels: 8 slow reps

1
Stand with your feet wider than your hips, and turn out your toes slightly. Place your hands on your hips, tilt your pelvis and lengthen your spine.

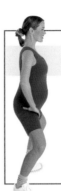

Don't forget...

Keep your pelvis tilted to prevent your bottom from pushing out. Ensure that your back is in a straight line as you bend; do not lean forwards.

2
Slowly bend your knees over your toes. Keep your spine lifted and your head up. Only bend as far as you feel comfortable without lifting your heels up from the floor. Now, pull in your abdominals and slowly straighten your knees, taking care not to lock them before repeating as recommended above.

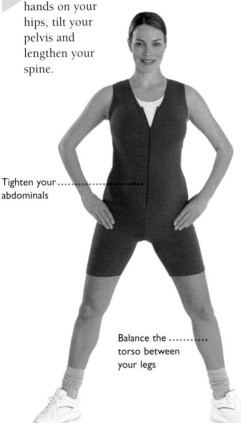

Tighten your abdominals

Balance the torso between your legs

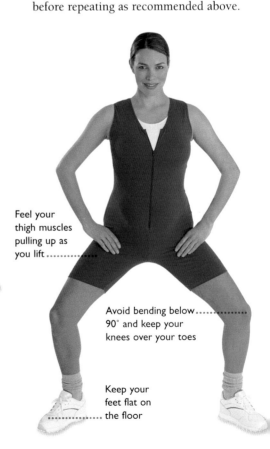

Feel your thigh muscles pulling up as you lift

Avoid bending below 90° and keep your knees over your toes

Keep your feet flat on the floor

CAUTION

If you experience discomfort around your pubic bone during this exercise, try reducing the width of your stance. If discomfort continues, you should omit this exercise.

Knee raise

To warm and loosen the hips and knees, and to increase your body temperature

GENTLE   MODERATE   ENERGETIC

All levels: 16 alternate reps (8 with each leg)

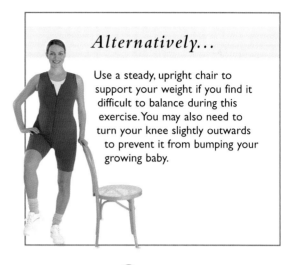

Alternatively...

Use a steady, upright chair to support your weight if you find it difficult to balance during this exercise. You may also need to turn your knee slightly outwards to prevent it from bumping your growing baby.

1

Stand tall with your feet hip-width apart. Tilt your pelvis and tighten your abdominals to support your baby and your back.

Keep your chest lifted and avoid leaning forwards towards your raised knee........

Ensure that your supporting foot is flat on the floor................

2

Lift your right knee to a comfortable height in front of you, keeping your back straight, abdominals tight and shoulders down. Make sure the supporting knee remains soft.

Place your hands on your hips for extra stability

Relax your toes

3

Lower your right leg back to the floor and repeat with the left leg. Lift out of the supporting hip each time you transfer your weight. When you feel ready, touch your hand to your opposite knee as it is raised. Continue for the recommended reps.

Replace your foot directly under your hip to prevent your pelvis from rocking

5

Chest opener

To expand your chest and to loosen your upper body

GENTLE   MODERATE   ENERGETIC

8 slow reps

1 Stand with your feet slightly more than hip-width apart and relax your arms by your sides. Tilt your pelvis and stand tall.

Tighten your abdominals

2 Lift up your arms to shoulder height. Don't lock out your elbows and remember to pull in your abdominals.

Try not to let your arms drop

Don't push out your chest

Ensure that your knees remain soft

3 Slowly round your back and curl forwards, bringing your arms slowly around to the front. Keep your head relaxed throughout.

Scoop your abdominals inwards to curl your spine

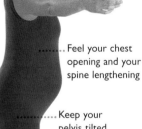

4 Lengthen your body as you open your arms out to the side, pulling the shoulder blades down and back together. Repeat as directed.

Feel your chest opening and your spine lengthening

Keep your pelvis tilted when returning your arms to the centre

Arm circles

To warm and loosen your shoulders and to open your chest

GENTLE   MODERATE   ENERGETIC

All levels: 8 reps with each arm

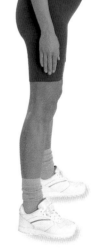

Stand with your feet just over hip-width apart and relax your arms by your sides.

Tighten your abdominals

Emphasize the full circular movement, paying particular attention to the backwards phase

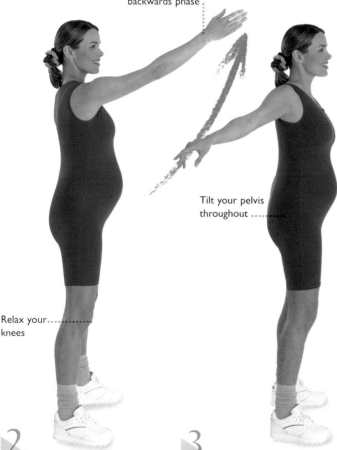

Press your shoulder firmly down on completion of each circular movement

Tilt your pelvis throughout

Relax your knees

2
With your hips and shoulders facing forwards, take the right arm around in a slow circle, starting with a forwards action.

3
Keeping the movement slow and continuous, take your right arm up close to your ear and then back as far as possible. During this backwards movement tighten the abdominals to avoid arching your back.

4
Finish the movement by lowering your arm in a slow controlled way, back down to your side again. Continue as directed, then repeat with your left arm.

Side bend

To warm and loosen your spine

GENTLE   MODERATE   ENERGETIC

All levels: 16 alternate reps (8 on each side)

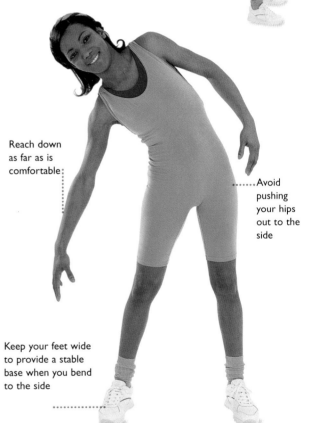

Don't forget...

Bring the leading arm slightly forwards as you bend to the side to prevent you from leaning back. This can place extra strain on your spine which may cause backache, especially during the second and third trimesters.

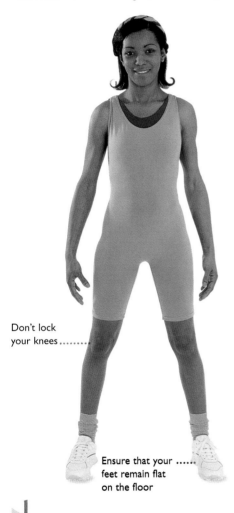

Don't lock
your knees ....

Ensure that your ......
feet remain flat
on the floor

Reach down
as far as is
comfortable

Avoid
pushing
your hips
out to the
side

Keep your feet wide
to provide a stable
base when you bend
to the side

1

Stand with your feet just over hip-width apart and relax your arms by your sides. Tilt your pelvis, pull in your abdominal muscles to support your back and lengthen your spine.

2

Bend slowly from the waist, reaching down sideways to the right. Tighten the abdominals, relax your shoulders and keep your chest open as you come up to the starting position. Repeat to the other side, then continue for the recommended reps.

Neck mobility

To release tension in your neck

GENTLE   MODERATE   ENERGETIC

All levels: 4 alternate reps (2 on each side)

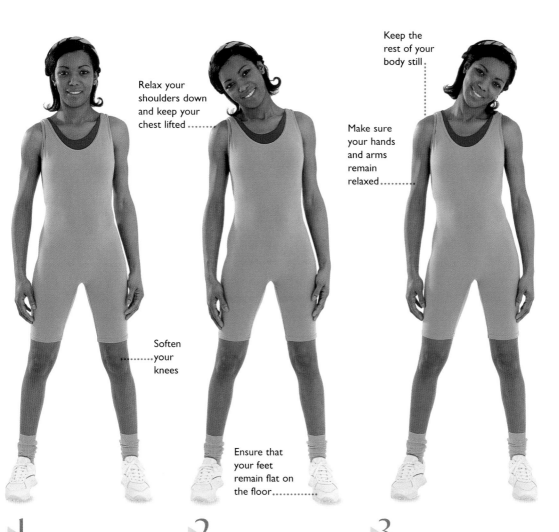

Relax your shoulders down and keep your chest lifted ....

Soften .... your knees

Keep the rest of your body still .

Make sure your hands and arms remain relaxed ....

Ensure that your feet remain flat on the floor............

1

Stand with your feet slightly wider than hip-width and relax your arms by your sides. Keep your shoulders down and lengthen your neck. Tilt your pelvis, tighten your abdominals to lift your baby and stand tall.

2

Keeping your shoulders relaxed, take your head gently over to the right side, pressing your ear towards the shoulder. Keep your shoulders down and pause.

3

Return your head to the centre, tighten the abdominals, tilt your pelvis and stand tall. Repeat to your left side, then continue as directed above.

Ankle mobility

To warm and loosen your ankles

GENTLE   MODERATE   ENERGETIC

All levels: 8 reps with each ankle

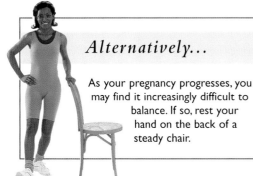

Alternatively...

As your pregnancy progresses, you may find it increasingly difficult to balance. If so, rest your hand on the back of a steady chair.

1 Stand with your feet a couple of inches apart, and place your hands on your hips for extra stability. Tilt your pelvis, tighten your abdominals and stand tall.

Ensure that your feet are flat on the floor

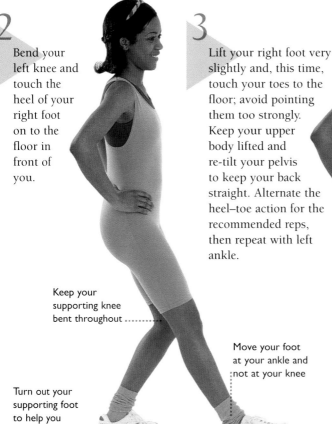

2 Bend your left knee and touch the heel of your right foot on to the floor in front of you.

Keep your supporting knee bent throughout

Turn out your supporting foot to help you balance

3 Lift your right foot very slightly and, this time, touch your toes to the floor; avoid pointing them too strongly. Keep your upper body lifted and re-tilt your pelvis to keep your back straight. Alternate the heel–toe action for the recommended reps, then repeat with left ankle.

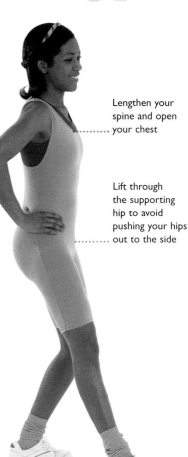

Lengthen your spine and open your chest

Lift through the supporting hip to avoid pushing your hips out to the side

Move your foot at your ankle and not at your knee

Foot mobility

To warm and loosen your ankles and feet and increase circulation to your feet

GENTLE   MODERATE   ENERGETIC

All levels: 8 reps with each foot

Alternatively...

As your pregnancy progresses, you may find it becomes increasingly difficult to maintain your balance, especially in the third trimester. If so, try resting your hand on the back of an upright, steady chair for support.

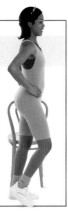

1

Stand with your feet a few inches apart. Place your hands on your hips, transfer your weight on to your right leg and lift through the right hip. Tilt your pelvis, tighten your abdominals to support your baby and stand tall.

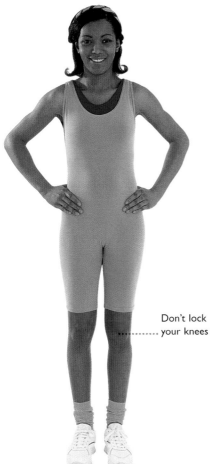

Don't lock your knees

2

Lift the heel of your left foot as high as possible, bending your foot at the toe joint and lifting through the arch of your foot. Lift up through your right hip to ensure that your hips are in line. Re-tilt your pelvis and re-tighten your abdominals. Pause, then lower your left heel back to the floor. Continue as directed, then repeat with your right foot.

Make sure your upper body is lifted and your chest is open

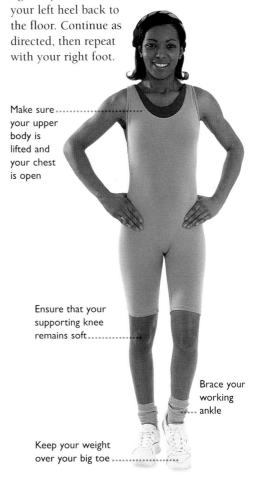

Ensure that your supporting knee remains soft

Brace your working ankle

Keep your weight over your big toe

Marching on the spot

To warm your muscles and increase circulation

GENTLE   MODERATE   ENERGETIC

Continue for 1–2 minutes until you feel warmer

1
Stand with your feet a few inches apart and relax your arms by your sides. Tighten your abdominals to support your baby and your back and stand tall.

2
March briskly on the spot, raising your knees up to a comfortable height.

3
Bend your arms at the elbows and move them forwards and backwards with each step. Make sure that your abdominals are tight and your chest is lifted. Continue as directed.

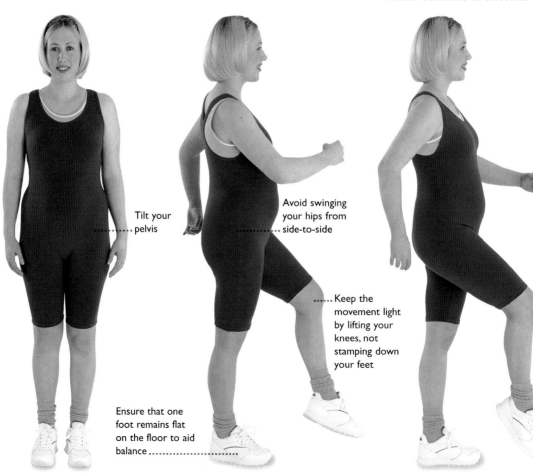

Tilt your pelvis

Avoid swinging your hips from side-to-side

Keep the movement light by lifting your knees, not stamping down your feet

Ensure that one foot remains flat on the floor to aid balance

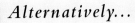

Calf stretch

*To stretch and lengthen the calf muscle. This can be
particularly helpful if you suffer from cramp*

GENTLE   MODERATE   ENERGETIC

All levels: Hold for a count of 8 on each side

Alternatively...

You may need some support for
this exercise, especially in the third
trimester. If so, stand sideways to
the back of a steady chair and
rest your hand on top of it, but
avoid leaning into the chair.

3

Bend your left knee until it
aligns with your left ankle and
gently press your right heel
into the floor. Re-tilt your
pelvis, lift your baby in
towards you and keep both
hips facing forwards. If you
cannot feel the stretch, move
your right foot further back.
Hold as directed,
then change
legs.

..... Tighten your
abdominals

Lean slightly ....
forwards with
your upper body
to maintain a
diagonal line from
your head to
back heel

.... Ensure that
your knees
remain soft

1

Stand with your feet
hip-width apart, place
your hands on your hips
and tilt the pelvis.

2

Keeping your feet wide and
toes facing forwards, take
a large step backwards
with your right foot.
Ensure that your
spine remains long
and chest is open.

.............Feel the stretch
in the bulky part
of your calf

Quadriceps stretch

To stretch and lengthen the muscles at the front of your thighs. These muscles often feel quite tight during pregnancy

GENTLE   MODERATE   ENERGETIC

Hold for a count of 8 on each side

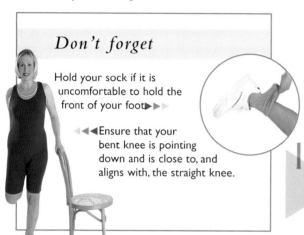

Don't forget

Hold your sock if it is uncomfortable to hold the front of your foot ▶▶

◀◀◀Ensure that your bent knee is pointing down and is close to, and aligns with, the straight knee.

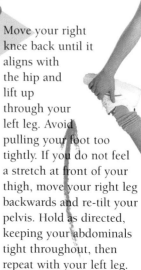

1 Stand with your left side to a chair and rest your left hand on the back of it for support. With your feet about hip-width apart, transfer your weight on to your left leg, lift through your left hip and tilt your pelvis.

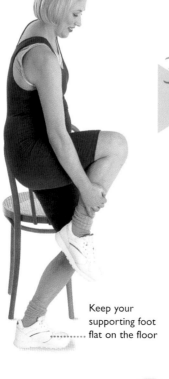

2 With your left leg bent, lift your right knee up in front of you and hold your ankle at the front.

Keep your supporting foot flat on the floor

3 Move your right knee back until it aligns with the hip and lift up through your left leg. Avoid pulling your foot too tightly. If you do not feel a stretch at front of your thigh, move your right leg backwards and re-tilt your pelvis. Hold as directed, keeping your abdominals tight throughout, then repeat with your left leg.

Side stretch

To stretch the latissimus dorsi and obliques, and to lengthen your spine

GENTLE   MODERATE   ENERGETIC

All levels: Hold for a count of 6 on each side; repeat if desired

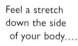

Don't forget...

Position your arm slightly forwards and keep your pelvis tilted to avoid arching your back. Be careful not to bend over too far if you feel any discomfort in your abdomen.

Relax your shoulders down

Ensure that you keep your upper arm stretched

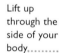

Lift up through the side of your body

Feel a stretch down the side of your body

Keep your weight central to avoid tipping your hips to the side

1
Stand with your feet wider than your hips and make sure your knees are soft. Place your hands on your hips and tilt your pelvis. Tighten your abdominals to lift your baby and stand tall.

2
Reach your right arm up to the ceiling just in front of your head and lengthen your spine.

3
Bend directly to the left, reaching your arm up and over to the side. Keep your abdominals tight and pelvis tilted. Hold as directed, then repeat on the other side.

Triceps stretch

To stretch and lengthen the muscles at the back of your upper arms

1

Stand with your feet slightly more than hip-width apart. Keep your knees soft and tighten your abdominals.

Keep your pelvis tilted

Don't forget...

◄◄◄ Ensure your head is lifted and in line with your spine.

If your back begins to arch, try supporting the arm with your other hand from the front. ►►►

GENTLE   MODERATE   ENERGETIC

Hold for a count of 8 on each side

2

Stand tall and lift your right arm towards the ceiling.

....Stretch your arm straight up above your head; ensure that you keep your elbow soft

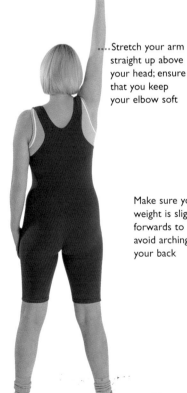

Make sure your.... weight is slightly forwards to avoid arching your back

3

Bend your right elbow so it points to the ceiling and reach down between your shoulder blades with your fingers.

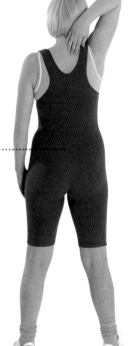

4

Take hold of your right elbow with your left hand and ease the elbow gently behind your head. Re-tilt your pelvis and tighten the abdominals to prevent your back from arching. Feel the stretch in the back of your right upper arm. Hold as directed, then repeat with your left arm.

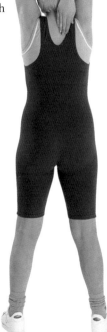

Hip stretch

To stretch and lengthen the hip flexors to improve your pelvic tilt

GENTLE   MODERATE   ENERGETIC

Hold for a count of 6 on each side

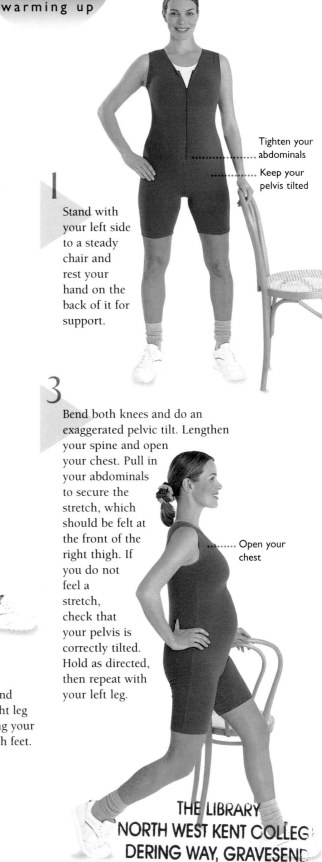

Tighten your abdominals

Keep your pelvis tilted

1 Stand with your left side to a steady chair and rest your hand on the back of it for support.

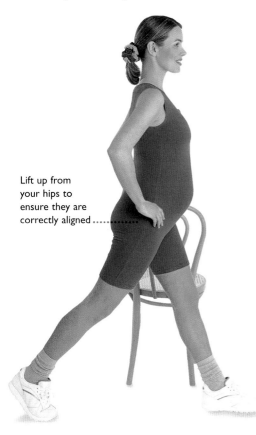

Lift up from your hips to ensure they are correctly aligned

3 Bend both knees and do an exaggerated pelvic tilt. Lengthen your spine and open your chest. Pull in your abdominals to secure the stretch, which should be felt at the front of the right thigh. If you do not feel a stretch, check that your pelvis is correctly tilted. Hold as directed, then repeat with your left leg.

Open your chest

2 With your feet wider than your hips and your toes facing forwards, step the right leg back. Lift the heel off the floor, keeping your weight evenly distributed between both feet. Lengthen your spine and stand tall.

Adductor stretch

To stretch and lengthen your inner thigh muscles

GENTLE   MODERATE   ENERGETIC

Hold for a count of 8 on each side

Alternatively...

As your pregnancy progresses, the extra weight of your growing baby may affect your ability to balance; if so, rest your hand on the back of a steady chair for support.

1

Stand with your feet as wide apart as is comfortable and turn your toes outwards. Place your hands on your hips and tilt your pelvis.

Tighten your abdominals to support your baby and your back

2

Keeping your right toes turned outwards, move your left foot so your toes face forwards. With your left leg straight, bend the right knee and transfer your weight over to the right side. Re-tilt your pelvis, lengthen your spine and open your chest. You may feel a mild ache in your right thigh as the muscles work hard to hold you in position. Hold as directed, then repeat on the other side.

CAUTION

Stop immediately if you experience any discomfort or pain at the front of your pelvis. First, try reducing the width of your feet when doing this exercise, but if this still feels uncomfortable omit this stretch from the workout.

Keep your knee in line with your ankle

Feel a stretch in the inner thigh of your straight leg

Ensure that both feet remain flat on the floor

Avoid rolling the ankle of the straight leg

Pectoral stretch

To stretch and lengthen your chest muscles which may feel tight and restricted. This stretch will help to improve your posture

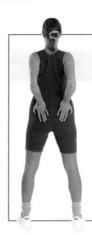

Don't forget...

Squeeze your shoulder blades together in order to feel the stretch across your chest and front of your shoulders. Ensure that your palms are rested on your buttocks (not on the hips) to gain maximum benefit from this exercise.

GENTLE   MODERATE   ENERGETIC

All levels: Hold for a count of 6; repeat if desired

1 Stand with your feet slightly wider than hip-width apart and keep your knees soft. Rest your hands just above your buttocks, tighten your abdominals to lift your baby and stand tall.

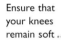

Ensure that your knees remain soft ....

Keep your weight evenly distributed over both feet ....

Lengthen your neck and keep it in line with your spine..............

Tighten your abdominals

2 Lift your chest and draw both elbows back, slowly squeezing your shoulder blades together. Keep your abdominals tight, to prevent your back from arching, and ensure that your neck and spine are aligned. Hold as directed; you should feel the stretch across your chest and the front of your shoulders.

Don't push forwards on to your toes or rock backwards on to your heels

COMMON MISTAKES

Arched spine You may be tempted to push your abdomen and chest out during this exercise, but this will cause your back to arch badly. To avoid this mistake, keep your pelvis tilted and hold in your abdominal muscles.

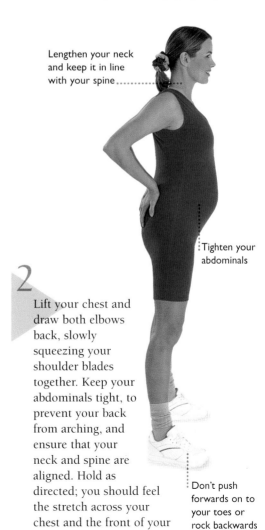

Upward reach

To stretch the latissimus dorsi and to lengthen your spine. This movement will increase the space in your abdomen and should help you to feel more comfortable

GENTLE   MODERATE   ENERGETIC

Hold for a count of 6 on each side; repeat if desired

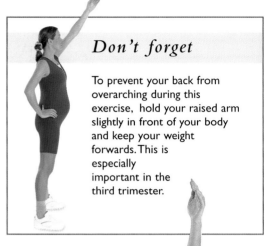

Don't forget

To prevent your back from overarching during this exercise, hold your raised arm slightly in front of your body and keep your weight forwards. This is especially important in the third trimester.

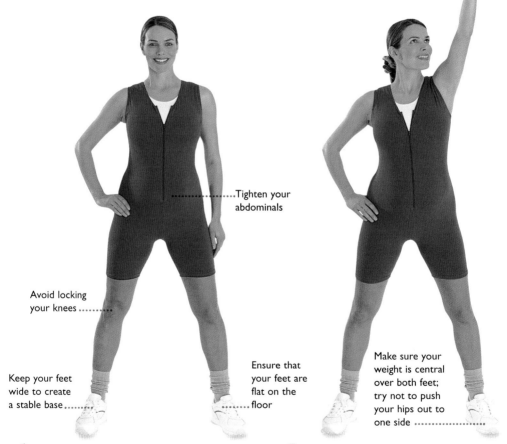

Tighten your abdominals

Avoid locking your knees

Keep your feet wide to create a stable base

Ensure that your feet are flat on the floor

Make sure your weight is central over both feet; try not to push your hips out to one side

1 Stand with your feet slightly more than hip-width apart and place your right hand on your hip. Tilt your pelvis, lengthen your spine and stand tall.

2 Keeping your head lifted, slowly reach up to the ceiling with your left arm. Lengthen your spine and extend the arm up as high as you can. Hold as directed above, then lower your arm. Relax your shoulders down, stand tall and repeat with the right arm.

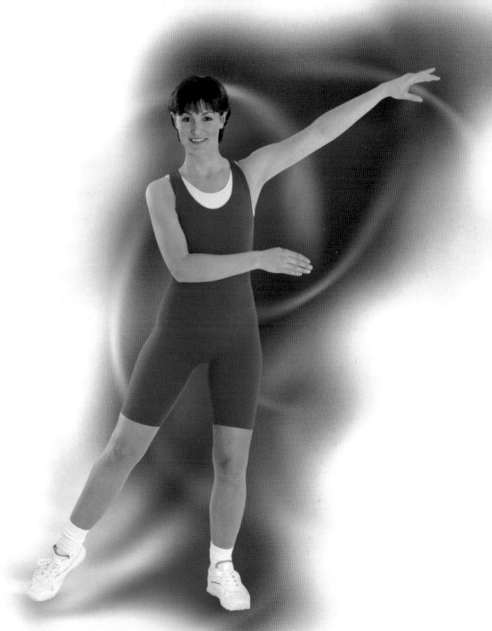

AEROBIC EXERCISE

*These easy-to-follow exercises provide a safe and effective aerobic workout appropriate for any stage of pregnancy. They have been specially selected so that you can complete them, unsupervised, in a relatively small space at home. During the exercises you should feel slightly out of breath, but still be able to hold a conversation. At the end of your session you should feel warm and invigorated, and will probably have a little more colour in your face. Try to keep your legs moving until your breathing has returned to normal and you are feeling cooler. And remember: you **must** always repeat the exercises in reverse order before stopping, take regular sips of water and exercise in a well-ventilated room.*

Double side step

GENTLE   MODERATE   ENERGETIC

16 alternate   *32 alternate*   *48 alternate*
double steps   *double steps*   *double steps*

FEELING ENERGETIC?

▶ Turn this into a travelling step by taking four steps to the right, then four steps to the left.

▶ Bend both knees as you join your feet together. But try to be careful not to lock them as you straighten your legs.

▶ Combine this exercise with one of the arm variations detailed on *page 24*.

1 Stand tall with your hands placed on your hips and your shoulders relaxed down. Tighten your abdominals to lift your baby and step out to the side to a comfortable width with your left foot.

Tilt your pelvis ....

Keep your...........
knees soft as
you step

2 Bring your right foot in to touch your left foot and then step to the left again. Repeat these two steps back to the right and continue as described. Keep your back straight and upper body lifted.

Tighten your ....
abdominals

Ensure that ....
your hips are
facing forwards
and are level
throughout

CAUTION

If you experience discomfort on or around the pubic bone, try taking narrower steps. If discomfort persists, however, omit this exercise.

Keep your feet low to the
ground to prevent this
movement from becoming
bouncy ....

Step touch

with "lift and lower"

Once you have mastered the foot movements, and provided that you have the energy, you can make the aerobic exercises more demanding by adding arm movements, which will work the upper body muscles. A further choice of arm movements is included on the following page.

GENTLE
16 alternate steps

MODERATE
24 alternate steps

ENERGETIC
32 alternate steps

Relax your shoulders

Control the arm movement; do not throw up your arms

1

With your feet together, tilt your pelvis and pull in your abdominals. Step to the side with your right foot, and as you do, lift your arms straight up to your sides to shoulder height. Relax your shoulders down and keep your back long.

Tighten your abdominals

Tilt your pelvis

2

Bring your left foot in to touch the side your right foot and, as you do, lower your arms down to your sides. Then, raise your arms again and repeat the movement to the left. Continue as recommended above.

arm variations

step touch with "biceps curl"

1

Keeping your elbows soft and fists lightly clenched, straighten your arms close to your body as you "step" out to the side.

2

Keeping your elbows close to your sides, bend your forearms up towards your shoulders as you "touch". Keep your chest lifted and shoulders relaxed.

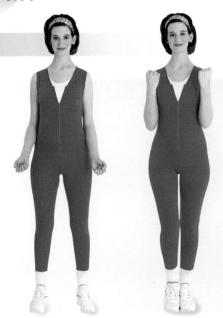

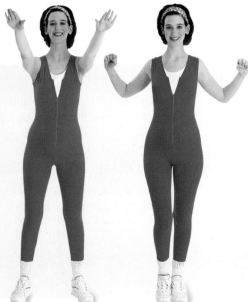

step touch with "high reach and pull"

1

Extend both arms forwards and up as you "step". Don't take the arms above your head as this could make your back arch.

2

With your fists lightly clenched, pull the arms down and back as you "touch". Squeeze your shoulder blades together and keep your abdominals pulled in.

step touch with "reach and pull"

1

Extend both arms forwards at shoulder height as you "step". Keep your elbows soft and shoulders relaxed.

2

With your fists lightly clenched, bend your elbows and pull both arms back as you "touch". Keeping your elbows high, squeeze your shoulder blades together.

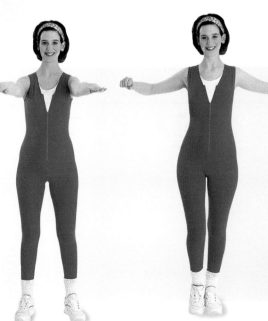

Heel digs

GENTLE	MODERATE	ENERGETIC
16 alternate digs	*16 alternate digs*	*32 alternate digs with "reach and pull"*

1

Stand with your feet wider than your hips and your knees soft. Tilt your pelvis and pull in the abdominals. Place your hands on the hips and transfer your weight on to your left foot. Stand tall, lift your chest and relax your shoulders down.

2

Bend the left knee and straighten the right leg out to the front, flexing your foot and touching the heel on to the floor. Keep your hips level and your pelvis tilted to prevent your back from overarching. Repeat with the other leg, then continue as directed.

..... Brace your ankle to keep your foot from rolling

Lift up through ..... the supporting hip to ensure that both hips are level

"Dig" the heel into the floor as ..... far away as possible

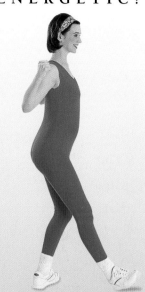

FEELING ENERGETIC?

► Add the "reach and pull" arm movement (*see page 24*).

► Bend the supporting knee deeper as you "dig" your heel *gently* into the floor.

► Add the "high reach and pull" arm movement (*see page 24*): start with both arms extended upwards and in front of you and then pull your elbows back as you *gently* "dig" your heel into the floor (*as above*).

Side taps

GENTLE	MODERATE	ENERGETIC
4 reps of 4 taps each side	8 reps of 4 taps each side	16 reps of 4 taps each side

FEELING ENERGETIC?

1

Stand with your feet together and place your hands on your hips. With your pelvis tilted, relax the shoulders down, lift your chest and lengthen your spine.

2

Bend your right knee and take your left leg out to the side, touching your toes on to the floor. Your weight should be on your right leg. Keep your hips level and your pelvis tilted to prevent your back from arching. Do four side taps with the left leg, then four with the right. Continue as directed.

▶ You can exercise your upper body by lifting both arms out to your sides at shoulder height with each side tap (*as above*).

▶ Bend the supporting knee deeper as you take your leg out to the side.

▶ Perform the "side taps" much slower and with more control in order to increase the aerobic intensity of this exercise.

Keep your hips level, particularly when you change legs

Ensure that your knees are soft

Ensure that the supporting knee is bent

Brace your ankles to keep your feet from rolling

"Tap" your foot out to the side as wide as possible

Knee raise

GENTLE	MODERATE	ENERGETIC
16 alternate raises	*32 alternate raises*	*32 alternate raises with "reach and pull"*

Pull in your abdominals to support your baby and your back

Ensure that you keep your knees soft

Replace your foot directly under the hip to prevent your hips rocking from side-to-side

Brace the supporting ankle to stop your foot from rolling

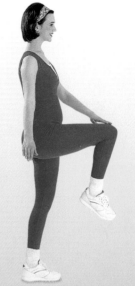

FEELING ENERGETIC?

▶ Raise your knee higher (*as above*), and lift your arms up to shoulder height before touching your opposite knee.

▶ Carefully bend the supporting knee as you lift your leg.

▶ Combine with the "reach and pull" arm movement (*see page 24*). With your arms at shoulder height, "pull" your arms back as you raise the knee, and "reach" as your lower it.

1

Stand with your feet about hip-width apart, relax your arms by your sides and tilt your pelvis.

2

Keeping your back straight, lift your right knee up to hip-height and touch it with your left hand. Lift your chest and relax your shoulders down. You may need to turn your knee slightly outwards to prevent it from bumping your abdomen. Lower your right knee, then repeat with your left leg, taking care to lift out of the supporting hip. Then, continue as directed.

Knee bend

with arm circles

Tilt your pelvis ....

Pull in your abdominals ....

CAUTION

If you experience discomfort around your pubic bone during this exercise, reduce the width of your stance. If discomfort continues omit this exercise.

1
Stand with your feet wider than hip-width apart and turn out your toes. Lift your arms up and out to the sides.

2
Keeping your heels down, bend your knees and slowly take your arms down in front of your body.

GENTLE   MODERATE   ENERGETIC

8 knee bends   *16 knee bends*   *24 knee bends*

Keep your body in a straight line .... as you bend

Tuck your bottom under ... as you bend

Stand tall.

Make sure .... your back is lifted

Feel the muscles in your thighs pulling up as .... you lift

Take care .... not to lock your knees as they straighten

3
When your bend is at its deepest, continue the arm circle, crossing your hands in front of your body.

4
Slowly straighten your knees and bring your arms up, continuing the large, circular movement.

5
Straighten your knees and open your arms out above you. Bring your arms down and repeat the sequence as recommended.

Bend and reach

GENTLE

16 alternate bends

MODERATE

32 alternate bends

ENERGETIC

32 alternate bends

Keep your pelvis tilted
.... throughout

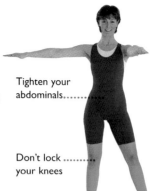

Tighten your abdominals.........

Don't lock ....
your knees

FEELING ENERGETIC?

- ► Try bending your knees a little deeper.
- ► Extend your front arm diagonally upwards.
- ► Push off from the extending leg to enlarge the movement.

1

Stand with your feet wider than hip-width and turn out your toes. Lift both arms out to the sides at shoulder height. As you bend both knees, bring your arms into your chest and keep your weight slightly forwards.

2

Straighten your knees, transfer your weight on to your right leg and touch your left foot out to the side, with your leg straight. At the same time, straighten your left arm out to the front and your right arm out to the side at shoulder height.

Keep your elbows lifted to shoulder height

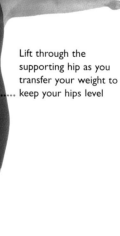

Lift through the supporting hip as you transfer your weight to
.... keep your hips level

Ensure that ....
your knees are over your toes as you bend

4

Transfer your weight on to your left leg, touch your right foot out, keeping you leg straight, and reverse the arm positions. Continue as directed.

3

Transfer your weight back to the centre, bend your knees and bring your arms back into your chest. Keep your neck long, shoulders down and chest lifted.

Single side step

with swinging arms

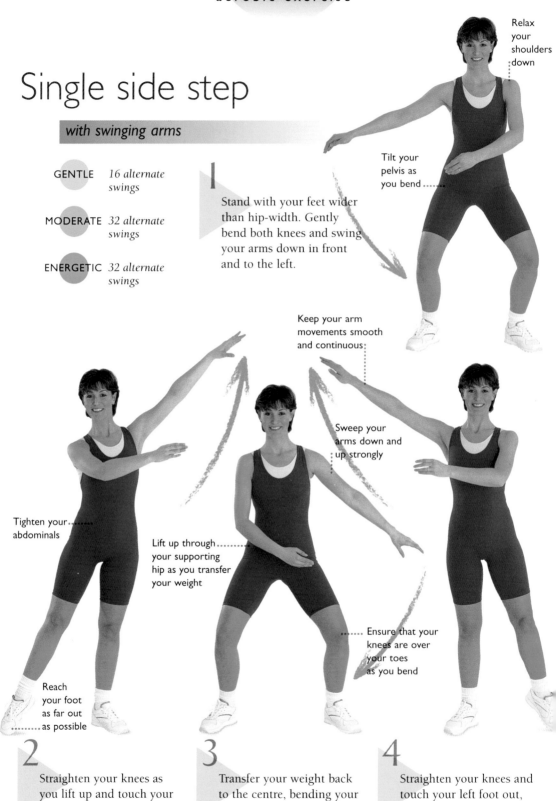

Relax your shoulders down

GENTLE   16 alternate swings

MODERATE 32 alternate swings

ENERGETIC 32 alternate swings

1 Stand with your feet wider than hip-width. Gently bend both knees and swing your arms down in front and to the left.

Tilt your pelvis as you bend

Keep your arm movements smooth and continuous

Sweep your arms down and up strongly

Tighten your abdominals

Lift up through your supporting hip as you transfer your weight

Ensure that your knees are over your toes as you bend

Reach your foot as far out as possible

2 Straighten your knees as you lift up and touch your right foot out to the side, swinging your arms high up to your left.

3 Transfer your weight back to the centre, bending your knees and bringing your arms back down as you do so.

4 Straighten your knees and touch your left foot out, this time bringing your arms up to the right. Continue as directed.

Travelling shuffle

GENTLE   MODERATE   ENERGETIC

Continue for   *Continue for*   *Continue for*
30 seconds   *1 minute*   *2 minutes*

FEELING ENERGETIC?

▶ Bend your knees further as you step to work your thigh muscles a little more.

▶ Take larger steps and make your arm movements bigger. Emphasize the backwards movement of your arms.

▶ Turn this exercise into a more continuous, travelling step by performing it in a large space.

1 Stand tall, with your feet a few inches apart. Hold your arms by your sides and clench your fists.

2 Step forwards with your right foot. Bend both knees and, with your elbows bent, bring your arms in front.

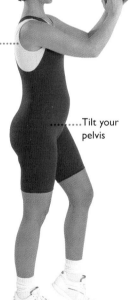

Lift and lengthen the spine as you bring your arms forwards..........

Lengthen your back at all times ....

Avoid thrusting your hips on the forwards step

..........Tilt your pelvis

3 Step the left foot in beside the right, bringing your elbows back in a shunting action. Keep your back lifted and relax your shoulders down.

Keep both feet flat on the floor when they are together..............

4 With both feet facing forwards, and your abdominals tight, repeat the step, keeping the arm movements large.

5 This time, bring the left foot in to touch only, and clap your hands up in front at shoulder height. Turn around and repeat with your left foot leading. Continue as directed.

Stride walk

GENTLE	MODERATE	ENERGETIC
Continue for 30 seconds	*Continue for 1 minute*	*Continue for 2 minutes*

Keep your elbows bent, gradually lifting them higher as you increase the pace

Make your stride as large as is comfortable

1 Walk around the room (or garden) with a bold, striding step. Keep your chest lifted and relax your shoulders.

Relax your shoulders down

Try to keep your head upright

Ensure that your weight is slightly forwards

Lift through the hips each time you step to avoid excessive rocking

Pull in your abdominals

4 March on the spot with your knees lifted to turn yourself around and continue as recommended. Try to keep your hips level and lightly touch your feet on the floor with each step.

Maintain a heel-toe action

2 Keeping your elbows bent, gradually lift them higher as you increase your pace. Remember to press your shoulders down.

3 Make sure your heel strikes the floor first and press down through your foot with each step. Keep your pelvis tilted and abdominals tight.

CAUTION

If you experience discomfort around your pubic bone during this exercise try reducing the length of your stride. If discomfort continues you should omit this exercise.

Touch back

1

Stand one pace back from a wall, lean slightly forwards and place the palms of your hands on the wall at shoulder height. Tilt your pelvis and tighten your abdominal muscles.

GENTLE	MODERATE	ENERGETIC
8 alternate touches	16 alternate touches	32 alternate touches

Squeeze your buttocks .... and stand tall as you begin and while you change legs

Lean your............. upper body forwards

2

Bend your right leg and *slowly* straighten your left leg out behind you, touching your toes on the floor; at the same time bring your upper body forwards to avoid arching your back. Return to the start position, tighten your buttocks and stand tall, then *slowly* bend your left leg and straighten out your right. Continue as directed.

.... Lift through the supporting hip, keeping both hips level and square to the wall

..... Bend your supporting knee

.........•....... Keep your back heel off the floor

Double side step

with circling arms

GENTLE	MODERATE	ENERGETIC
8 alternate double steps	*16 alternate double steps*	*16 alternate double steps*

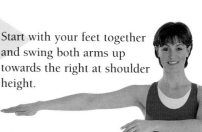

1 Start with your feet together and swing both arms up towards the right at shoulder height.

Tighten your........... abdominals to support your baby and your back

2 Keeping your hips square and level, step out to the left and gently bend both knees while beginning to circle your arms down. Keep your pelvis tilted.

Bend your knees further to make the exercise more demanding

Make sure that the movement is smooth and continuous, and as large as possible ....

Keep your arms slightly forwards during the upward movement to prevent your back from arching

3 Continue to swing your arms round and up to the left as you transfer your weight on to your left leg. Remember to lift up through your spine; feel a stretch down your right side.

Keep your hips level and facing forwards

4 Close your right foot in beside the left, taking your arms above your head. Now, take another step to the left, circling your arms down and around to the left once again. Finish with your weight on your left leg, your right foot touching on the floor and your arms up to the ceiling. Pause, lengthen your spine and open your chest before repeating the sequence to the right. Continue as recommended.

Step ups

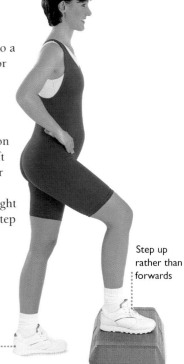

GENTLE

Continue for 30 seconds

MODERATE

Continue for 1 minute

ENERGETIC

Continue for 2 minutes

1 Stand close to a step block (or the bottom step of a flight of stairs). Rest your hands on your hips, lift through your left hip, and place your right foot on the step block.

Step up rather than forwards

Stay close to the step

2 Tilt your pelvis, pull in your abdominals, and step up with your right foot, keeping your hips level and your weight slightly forwards. Lift your chest and relax your shoulders down.

3 Keeping your back and chest lifted and pelvis tilted, bring your left foot up on to the block, next to the right foot.

Keep your head up and in line with your spine

4 Step down with your right foot first and touch the left foot in beside. Repeat with your left leg leading and continue as recommended.

Lift through the supporting hip with each step

Do not rock your hips from side-to-side

Keep your steps slow and rhythmic

Keep your knees soft as they straighten

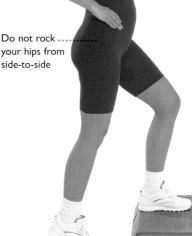

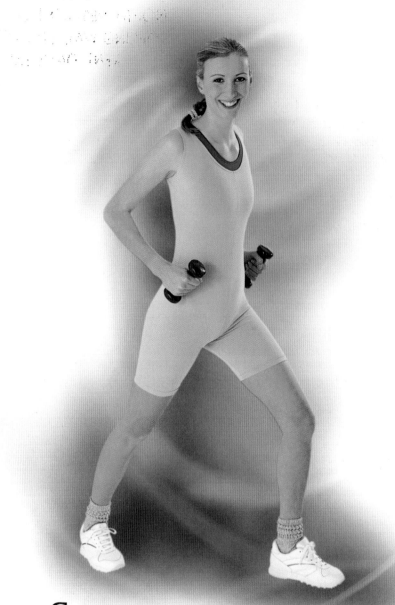

STRENGTHENING AND TONING

These exercises increase the strength and endurance of your muscles, thereby improving your posture, making daily tasks easier to perform and increasing your metabolic rate. Muscles that are not exercised will shrink and appear flabby, while trained muscles will be firmer. I have specially selected each exercise to target individual muscles which require increased strength for pregnancy and beyond. To make sure these exercises are effective, you should repeat the exercise again after a short break. You can use small weights or a resistance band to increase the intensity, if desired.

Standing gluteal raise

*To strengthen your buttock muscles, which
will help with bending and lifting*

GENTLE   MODERATE   ENERGETIC

2 sets of 8 reps   *2 sets of 16 reps*   *3 sets of 16 reps*
with each leg   *with each leg*   *with each leg*

Up to 28 weeks...

…you can do this exercise
kneeling but be careful not
to let your back arch and
avoid this if you feel
nauseous or suffer from
heartburn.

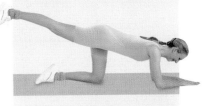

▶ Kneel on all fours with
your forearms under your
shoulders.

▶ Keeping your head and
spine aligned, extend one
leg and lift it as high as
you can behind you.
Lower, repeat, then
switch legs.

1 Stand one pace back from a
wall with your feet facing
forwards about hip-width
apart. Bend slightly
forwards and place your
hands on the wall at
shoulder height. Lengthen
your right leg out behind,
keeping your toes on the
floor. Lift through your left
hip to keep the hips level.

2 Keeping your upper body
forwards and both hips
parallel to the wall, squeeze
your buttocks and slowly
lift your right leg to a
comfortable height behind
you. Slowly lower your leg
to the floor and pull up out
of your left hip. Continue
as directed, then repeat
with your left leg.

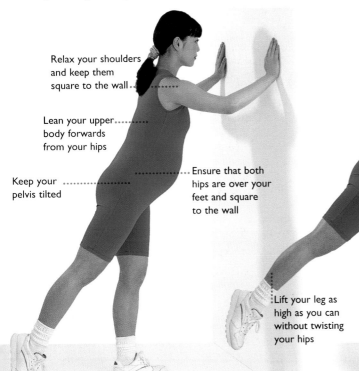

Relax your shoulders
and keep them
square to the wall

Lean your upper
body forwards
from your hips

Keep your
pelvis tilted

Ensure that both
hips are over your
feet and square
to the wall

Lift your leg as
high as you can
without twisting
your hips

Tighten your
abdominals

Take a short break if
your supporting hip
begins to ache

CAUTION

Keep your upper body
forwards and don't lift your
leg too high as this causes
stress to the lower back;
controlled movement is
essential.

Standing hamstring curl

*To strengthen the muscles at the back of your thighs,
which will help with bending and lifting*

GENTLE	MODERATE	ENERGETIC
2 sets of 8 reps with each leg	*2 sets of 16 reps with each leg*	*3 sets of 16 reps with each leg*

1 Stand one pace back from a wall with your feet hip-width apart. Bend slightly forwards and place your hands on the wall at shoulder height. Take the right leg out behind and lengthen it away from you. With your upper body forwards, flex the right foot and lift your right leg.

2 Keeping your thigh lifted and hips square to the wall, bend your right knee and draw the heel in towards your buttock. Straighten out your knee and continue as directed.

Up to 28 weeks...

...you can do this exercise kneeling but do not arch your back, and omit if you feel nauseous or suffer from heartburn.

▶ Kneel on all fours with your forearms under your shoulders.

▶ Keeping your head and spine in line, extend one leg, bend the knee and lift it as high as you can; lower, repeat, then switch legs.

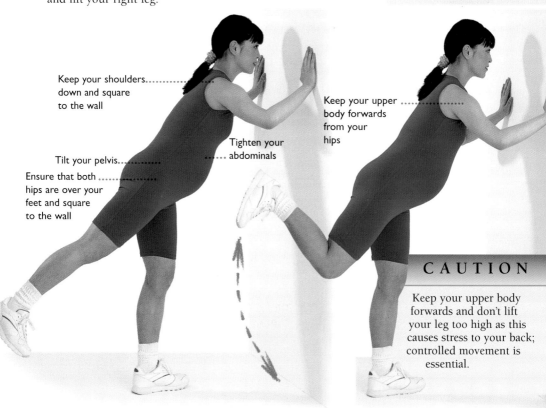

Keep your shoulders down and square to the wall

Tilt your pelvis

Ensure that both hips are over your feet and square to the wall

Tighten your abdominals

Keep your upper body forwards from your hips

CAUTION

Keep your upper body forwards and don't lift your leg too high as this causes stress to your back; controlled movement is essential.

Forward lunge

To strengthen the quadriceps (muscles at the front of your thighs) and the gluteals (buttock muscles), which will help with bending and lifting

GENTLE

2 sets of 8 reps with each leg

MODERATE

2 sets of 16 reps with each leg

ENERGETIC

3 sets of 16 reps with each leg

Alternatively...

This exercise is quite demanding, so only bend a little way at first. You can bend lower when your legs feel stronger. If you find this exercise ncomfortable or too strenuous on your knees, repeat the knee bends from the warm-up (see page 4).

1 Stand with your left side to a chair and rest your left hand on the back of it for support. With your feet hip-width apart and facing forwards, step your right leg back and lift your right heel off the floor; ensure that your weight is central between both feet. Tilt your pelvis and stand tall.

.... Tighten your abdominals

2 Keeping your back upright and abdominals tight, slowly bend both knees lowering your right knee towards the floor. Keep your left knee in line with your left ankle and your right knee in line with your right hip. Slowly push up to the starting position but don't lock out your knees. Re-tilt your pelvis and tighten your abdominals. Repeat as directed, then change sides.

Lengthen your spine and open ..... your chest

Keep your front knee over your ankle

The lower you bend the harder the exercise becomes ....

Leg extension

To strengthen the quadriceps (muscles at the front of your thighs) and to help to support your knees

GENTLE	MODERATE	ENERGETIC
2 sets of 8 reps with each leg	*2 sets of 16 reps with each leg*	*3 sets of 16 reps with each leg*

Alternatively...

You may find this exercise more comfortable to do sitting in a chair: sit upright in a straight-backed chair (or place a cushion behind your back for support) and slowly bend and straighten each leg; incorporate this into your office schedule!

1

Stand sideways to a chair and rest your left hand on the back of it for support. With your feet slightly apart and your right hand resting on your hip, transfer your weight on to your left leg and lift through your hip. With your pelvis tilted and your abdominals pulled in, lift your right knee off the floor to a comfortable height.

2

Keeping your thigh lifted, slowly straighten your right leg, but don't lock out your knee. Then, bend your knee back again, making sure your thigh remains lifted. Continue for the recommended reps, then lower your right leg, pulling up out of your left hip to keep the hips level. Repeat with your left leg.

Ensure that your thigh remains lifted as you straighten your leg

Keep your supporting knee soft

Brace your supporting ankle

Relax your toes

Calf raise

To strengthen the calf muscle and to increase the circulation in your legs. This exercise is particularly helpful if you have varicose veins

GENTLE

2 sets of 8 reps

MODERATE

2 sets of 16 reps

ENERGETIC

3 sets of 16 reps

1

Stand one pace back from a wall with your feet a few inches apart and your knees soft. Keeping your spine long, move your body weight slightly forwards, rest your hands lightly on the wall and look straight ahead.

2

Keeping your toes facing forwards and your weight distributed evenly between both feet, slowly rise up on to your toes. Ensure that your weight is forwards over your big toes and your chest is lifted. Lengthen your spine as you lift and keep your abdominals tight. Hold, then slowly lower both heels to touch lightly on the floor. Repeat as directed.

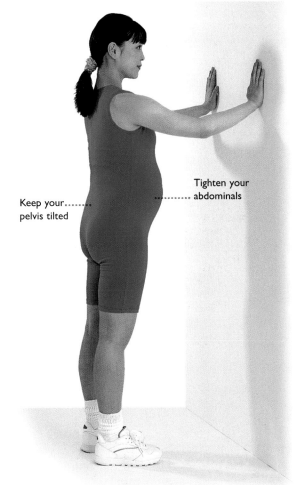

Keep your pelvis tilted

Tighten your abdominals

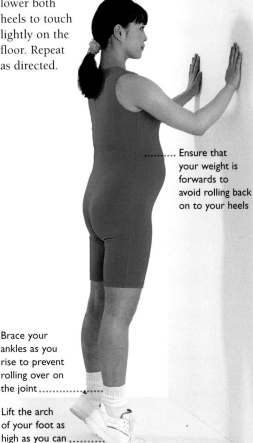

Ensure that your weight is forwards to avoid rolling back on to your heels

Brace your ankles as you rise to prevent rolling over on the joint

Lift the arch of your foot as high as you can

Biceps curl

To strengthen the muscles in the front of your upper arms, which will assist with lifting and carrying

GENTLE

2 sets of 8 reps

MODERATE

2 sets of 16 reps

ENERGETIC

3 sets of 16 reps

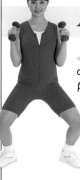

Alternatively...

◄◄◄ This exercise can be combined with a knee bend (see page 4). Stand with your feet wider than your hips. As you bend your knees, curl both arms up towards the shoulders with control. Lower your arms as you straighten your legs.

You may find this exercise more comfortable to perform sitting in a chair, provided there is sufficient room for your arms to straighten fully. Sit upright on a sturdy chair, or place a cushion behind your back for support, and slowly lift and lower both arms, keeping your wrists and forearms in line. ▶▶▶

CAUTION

If you feel light-headed after a few reps, combine this exercise with a knee bend or try the seated version (*see box, right*). Avoid leaning back as you raise your arms.

1

Stand with your feet slightly wider than your hips and keep your knees soft. Rest your arms by your sides with your elbows straight, but not locked, and hold a small weight firmly in each hand. With your palms facing in towards your body, tilt your pelvis, tighten your abdominals and stand tall.

2

Keeping your elbows firmly into your side, and your wrists and forearms in line, *slowly* curl your arms up towards the shoulders. Keep your chest lifted and make sure your shoulders are relaxed down and back. Slowly lower the arms with resistance to the starting position, taking care not to let your elbows lock out. Pause, then repeat for the recommended reps.

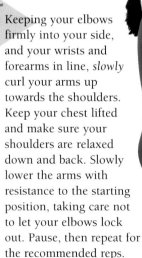

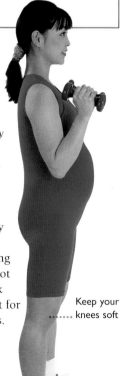

Keep your .... knees soft

Ensure that your weight is balanced .... between both feet

Pelvic floor exercises

To strengthen the muscles of your pelvic floor, which support your baby and reduce the risk of stress incontinence during and after pregnancy

GENTLE

MODERATE

ENERGETIC

Slow: 4 sets of 4 reps;
Fast: 4 sets of 6 reps

You can perform these exercises in any position – lying, standing, or sitting – without it being visible to anyone else, so try to do them as often as possible – at work, in the car, or watching television. Do *not*, however, perform this exercise while you are urinating as it may cause infection.

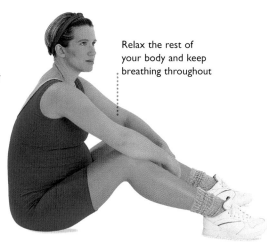

1

Slow contractions Stand, lie or sit with your feet slightly apart. Draw up and tighten the muscles around the anal sphincter; then hold. Slowly tighten the muscles around the urinary sphincter as well and lift up through the vagina. Hold for a count of 6, release with control, then repeat as recommended above right. If you've never worked these muscles, it may be difficult to isolate the movements individually, but it will get easier with practice.

Relax the rest of your body and keep breathing throughout

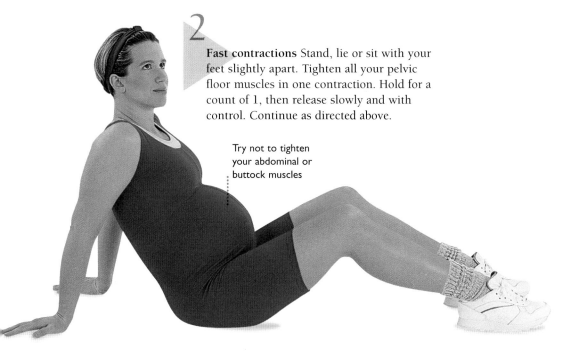

2

Fast contractions Stand, lie or sit with your feet slightly apart. Tighten all your pelvic floor muscles in one contraction. Hold for a count of 1, then release slowly and with control. Continue as directed above.

Try not to tighten your abdominal or buttock muscles

FIRST TRIMESTER ONLY

Lying pelvic tilt

To keep your back in correct alignment and to exercise the abdominals

GENTLE

2 sets of 8 reps

MODERATE

2 sets of 16 reps

ENERGETIC

3 sets of 16 reps

COMMON MISTAKES

Arched spine Make sure that your back remains in contact with the floor throughout this exercise. You may be tempted to arch your spine when you release the pelvic tilt, but this can cause back pain.

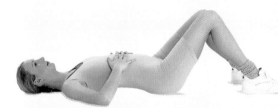

1 Lie on your back with your knees bent up and your feet flat on the floor, slightly less than hip-width apart. Relax your arms.

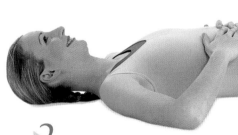

2 Lift your pubic bone gently upwards and feel the small of your back lightly touching the floor. Tighten your abdominal muscles and hold for a count of 6; keep breathing throughout. Release with control, then repeat as directed below.

Keep your knees bent and your feet flat on the floor

Feel your abdomen scooping in towards your spine

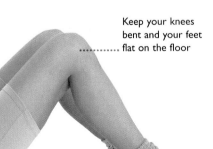

Keep your buttocks relaxed and in contact with the floor

FIRST TRIMESTER ONLY

Head and shoulder raise

To strengthen your abdominal muscles,
which support your baby and your back

GENTLE	MODERATE	ENERGETIC
2 sets of 8 reps	2 sets of 16 reps	3 sets of 16 reps

COMMON MISTAKES

Neck strain Make sure that there is plenty of space between your chin and your chest in order to avoid placing strain on your neck. If your head begins to feel heavy, place one hand behind your head to support your neck.

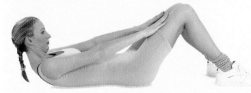

1

Lie on your back with your knees bent up and your feet flat on the floor, slightly less than hip-width apart. Place your hands on your thighs, tilt your pelvis and tighten your abdominals.

2

Keeping your abdomen firmly pulled in, breathe out and slowly raise your head and shoulders off the floor, sliding your hands up towards your knees. Leave a space between your chin and your chest as you lift. Keep the abdominals tight and breathe in as you lower. Keep your pelvis tilted and continue for the recommended reps at a controlled and steady pace.

CAUTION

Only raise your head and shoulders to the point where your abdomen can be held flat. If it begins to push out, ensure that you keep the curl lower.

Ensure that your neck is long and your shoulders remain down

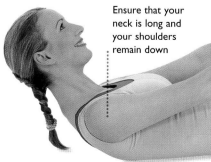

Keep your abdomen pulled in and flat

FIRST TRIMESTER ONLY
Lying abdominal lift

To strengthen your abdominal muscles, which help to support your baby and your back

GENTLE   MODERATE   ENERGETIC

All levels: 2 sets of 8 reps

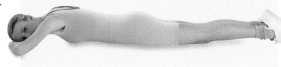

Alternatively...

If your breasts feel uncomfortable lying down, try this exercise kneeling on all fours. Keeping your hands under your shoulders and your neck and back aligned, pull your abdominals up towards your spine. Hold, then release with control.

1 If it is comfortable, lie on your front with your head turned to one side and your cheek resting on your hands. Relax your abdominals.

Keep your legs long and relaxed throughout

Try not to squeeze your buttocks

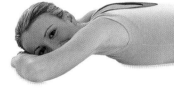

Feel your abdomen hollowing and lifting up toward your back

2 Now, lift your abdomen off the floor and squeeze it up in towards your spine; avoid tightening your buttocks or tilting your pelvis and keep your upper body relaxed. Hold for a count of 6, then release with control, letting your abdomen relax into the floor. Keep breathing throughout and continue for the recommended sets and reps.

COMMON MISTAKES

Back strain It may be tempting to lift your chest off the floor during this exercise in order to reduce the pressure on your breasts. Avoid this, however, as it can cause your back to overarch.

Kneeling abdominal lift

To strengthen your abdominal muscles, which help to support your baby and your back

GENTLE   MODERATE   ENERGETIC

All levels: 2 sets of 8 reps

1

Kneel on all fours, with your hands directly beneath your shoulders, your fingers facing forwards and your knees under your hips. Soften your elbows slightly and keep your back and neck long. Let your abdomen relax, but be careful not to let your back arch.

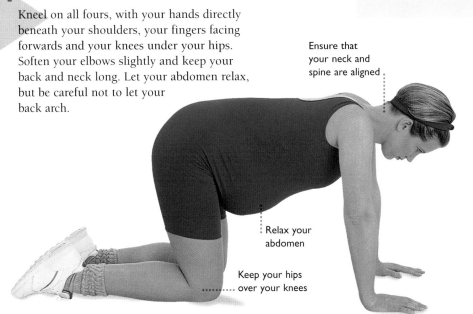

Ensure that your neck and spine are aligned

Relax your abdomen

Keep your hips over your knees

2

Breathe out and pull in your abdominals, lifting your baby in towards your spine. Keeping your elbows slightly bent, hold for a count of 6; remember to continue breathing. Lower your abdominals with control and relax your abdomen. Repeat as recommended above.

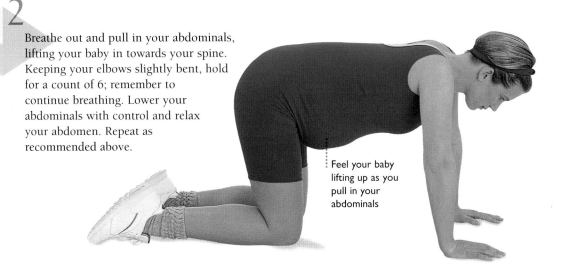

Feel your baby lifting up as you pull in your abdominals

Kneeling abdominal curl

To strengthen your abdominal muscles, which help to support your baby and your back

COMMON MISTAKES

Arched spine Do not let the weight of your abdomen and breasts pull your back down and arch your spine when you uncurl your body.

Alternatively...

If you find this position uncomfortable due to tingling or numbness in the fingers, you could try resting your elbows on the seat of a sturdy chair.

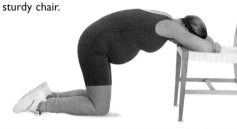

1 Kneel on all fours, with your hands directly beneath your shoulders, your fingers facing forwards and your knees under your hips. Keep your back and neck long and pull in the abdominals to prevent your back arching.

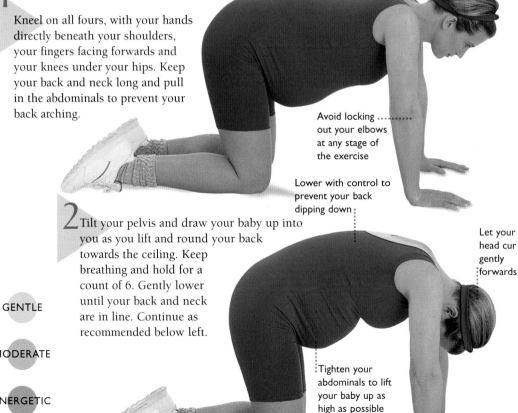

Avoid locking out your elbows at any stage of the exercise

Lower with control to prevent your back dipping down

2 Tilt your pelvis and draw your baby up into you as you lift and round your back towards the ceiling. Keep breathing and hold for a count of 6. Gently lower until your back and neck are in line. Continue as recommended below left.

Let your head cur gently forwards

GENTLE

MODERATE

ENERGETIC

Tighten your abdominals to lift your baby up as high as possible

All levels: 2 sets of 8 reps

Abdominal tightening

To strengthen your abdominal muscles, which support your baby and help you to maintain correct posture

GENTLE   MODERATE   ENERGETIC

All levels: 2 sets of 8 reps

1

Sit on an upright, sturdy chair (this exercise can also be performed standing or seated on the floor) and place some cushions behind your back for extra support. Relax your shoulders and place your arms by your sides.

2

Tighten your abdominals and lift your baby up and in towards you. Hold for a count of 6, then gently release; continue to breathe throughout. Repeat as directed. If your muscles begin to ache, rest before continuing.

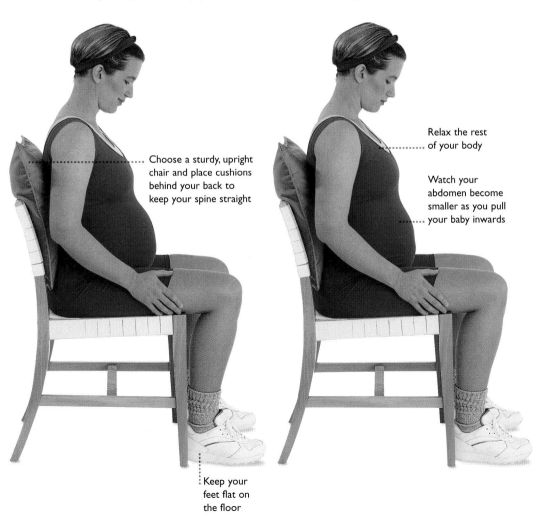

Choose a sturdy, upright chair and place cushions behind your back to keep your spine straight

Relax the rest of your body

Watch your abdomen become smaller as you pull your baby inwards

Keep your feet flat on the floor

49

Press up

To strengthen the pectorals (chest muscles), which support your breasts, and to tone the triceps (muscles in the back of your arms), which assist with lifting and carrying

1

Kneel on all fours, with your hands wider than your shoulders, your fingers facing forwards and your knees under your hips. With your neck in line with your spine, lengthen your back and tighten your abdominals.

Ensure that your body weight remains over your hands ....

2

Bend your elbows and lower your face towards the floor. Keep your head and spine aligned, your elbows over your wrists and your weight forwards as you *slowly* push up to the starting position; don't lock out your elbows. Repeat for the sets and reps recommended below.

Tighten your abdominals to prevent your back from arching.

GENTLE   *2 sets of 4 reps*   MODERATE   *2 sets of 8 reps*   ENERGETIC   *2 sets of 16 reps*

Alternatively...

This exercise will become more demanding as your baby grows. If you feel light-headed in the kneeling position, experience heartburn, discomfort in your knees or tingling in your fingers you should try the seated chest press instead. This version could even be included in your daily office schedule!

◄◄◄ Choose a sturdy chair with an upright back or place a cushion behind you for support. Tilt your pelvis, lift your chest and tighten the abdominals to support your baby and your back. Press your elbows together in front of your chest at shoulder height. If your breasts begin to feel uncomfortable, try leaving your elbows slightly apart.

Keeping your arms high, open your elbows out to the sides without arching your back. Keep your wrists and forearms in line as you bring both arms back in front of you. If you wish, hold a resistance band across your upper back with your arms out to the sides at shoulder height. Cross your arms in front of your chest, then open your arms out to your sides. ►►►

Shoulder shrug

To strengthen the trapezius (upper back muscles), which will help to improve your upper body posture

CAUTION

If you feel light-headed after a few repetitions you should combine this with a knee bend (*see page 4*) or follow the seated alternative (*see box, right*).

Alternatively...

If you prefer, you can do this exercise while sitting in a chair. Try to choose one with a straight back so you are able to sit upright, or place a cushion behind your back for extra support. This version could easily be incorporated into your everyday office schedule!

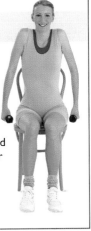

GENTLE *2 sets of 8 reps*   **MODERATE** *2 sets of 16 reps*   **ENERGETIC** *3 sets of 16 reps*

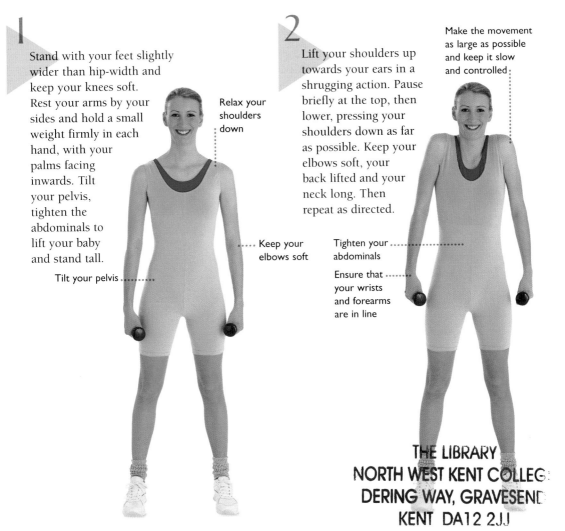

1 Stand with your feet slightly wider than hip-width and keep your knees soft. Rest your arms by your sides and hold a small weight firmly in each hand, with your palms facing inwards. Tilt your pelvis, tighten the abdominals to lift your baby and stand tall.

Relax your shoulders down

Tilt your pelvis

Keep your elbows soft

2 Lift your shoulders up towards your ears in a shrugging action. Pause briefly at the top, then lower, pressing your shoulders down as far as possible. Keep your elbows soft, your back lifted and your neck long. Then repeat as directed.

Make the movement as large as possible and keep it slow and controlled

Tighten your abdominals

Ensure that your wrists and forearms are in line

Shoulder squeeze

To strengthen the trapezius (upper back muscles), which will help to keep your shoulders back and improve your upper body posture

GENTLE

2 sets of 16 reps

MODERATE

3 sets of 16 reps

ENERGETIC

2 sets of 16 reps using resistance band

Alternatively...

◄◄◄ To make this exercise harder, try holding a resistance band in front of you at chest height. Then, keeping your hands slightly apart, squeeze your shoulder blades together.

You may find this exercise more comfortable to perform while kneeling on a mat or towel. Tilt your pelvis, keep your back straight and slowly squeeze your shoulder blades together. Ensure that your abdominals are pulled in to prevent your back from over-arching. ►►►

Ensure that the movement comes from the shoulders not the arms ....

Feel the muscles .... between your shoulder blades working

Pull in your .... abdominals

Ensure that ...... your knees remain soft

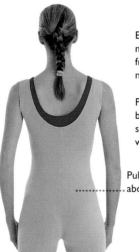

CAUTION

If you begin to feel light-headed after a few repetitions of this exercise, it is advisable to march on the spot (see page 12) or side step (see page 22) during this exercise – or follow the kneeling alternative (see above).

1 Stand with your feet slightly wider than your hips and keep your knees soft. Relax your arms by your sides. Tilt your pelvis and stand tall.

2 Pull your shoulders back, squeezing your shoulder blades together. Keep your spine long, your shoulders pressed down, and your abdominals tight to prevent your back from arching. Pause, return to the starting position and repeat as directed.

FIRST TRIMESTER ONLY

Lying pectoral press

To strengthen your chest muscles, which help to support your breasts and assist with lifting and carrying

GENTLE	MODERATE	ENERGETIC
sets of 8 reps	2 sets of 16 reps	3 sets of 16 reps

COMMON MISTAKES

Arched spine Keep your abdominal muscles tight to prevent your spine from overarching as you lower your arms to the floor. This will help to avoid backache and muscle spasms.

1 Lie on your back with your knees bent up and your feet flat on the floor. Tilt your pelvis and tighten your abdominals. With your shoulders relaxed, rest your arms on the floor and out to the side at shoulder height. Bend your elbows to 90°, keeping your forearms on the floor and the palms of your hands facing inwards.

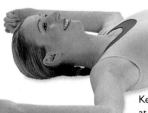

Keep your elbows bent at a 90° angle

If your breasts feel uncomfortable, keep your elbows slightly apart

Tighten your abdominals to prevent your back from arching during the lowering phase

Tilt your pelvis

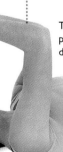

2 Slowly lift up your arms and press your elbows and forearms together above the chest. Keep your shoulders down and your neck long. Lower your arms with control, placing the whole arm on the floor at a 90° angle. Keep breathing as you repeat as recommended above.

CAUTION

If you feel dizzy or nauseous during this exercise it is recommended that you avoid lying on your back during your workout. Try the seated chest press or kneeling press up instead (see page 50).

Outer thigh raise

To strengthen the gluteals (buttock and outer thigh muscles), which help to stabilize your pelvis

GENTLE	MODERATE	ENERGETIC
2 sets of 8 reps with each leg	*2 sets of 16 reps with each leg*	*3 sets of 16 reps with each leg*

Alternatively...

If the knee of your top leg begins to feel uncomfortable, try bending your top knee slightly. Keep your weight forwards and perform the movement slowly.

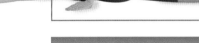

1

Lie on your right side, rest your head on your right arm and bend your right leg, keeping your knee slightly forwards. (Place a cushion under your abdomen if you wish.) Straighten the left leg, flex the foot and rotate the leg forwards so your toes are angled down towards the floor. With your pelvis tilted, lean slightly forwards and place your left hand on the floor in front of you.

CAUTION

Stop immediately if you begin to experience pain at the front or back of your pelvis. If the exercise feels uncomfortable in these areas, check your technique. If discomfort persists, omit this exercise.

Rotate the top hip forwards; do not roll back

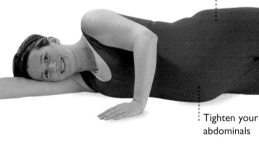

Tighten your abdominals

2

Lengthen the left leg away from the hip and slowly lift it, keeping your hip rotated forward, your foot flexed and your knee soft. Then, lower *slowly* and with control – do not allow your leg to drop suddenly; and keep breathing. Continue as directed, then switch legs.

Keep your pelvis tilted and pull in your abdominals to prevent your back from arching

Perform slowly ar carefully – don't b tempted to throw the leg up

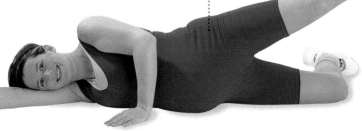

Inner thigh raise

*To strengthen the adductors (inner thigh muscles), which
will help to stabilize your pelvis*

GENTLE	MODERATE	ENERGETIC
2 sets of 8 reps with each leg	2 sets of 16 reps with each leg	3 sets of 16 reps with each leg

Alternatively...

If the knee joint of your
lower leg feels
uncomfortable as you lift it,
bend the knee slightly. Keep
your weight forwards and
lift and lower the leg *slowly*
and with control.

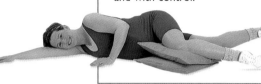

CAUTION

If you start to experience any
pain or discomfort in or around
your pelvis, you *must* omit this
exercise from your exercise programme.

1

Lie on your right side with your head resting
on your right arm. Bend your left leg
forwards and place your left knee on a couple
of cushions to keep it level with your hips.
Rest your left hand on the floor in front of
you for support and straighten your right leg
so that your right inner thigh faces upwards.

Tilt your pelvis
a little further if
your lower hip
is digging into
the floor

Tighten your
abdominals

2

Tilt your pelvis, tighten your abdominals and
lengthen your right leg away from your hip. Flex
your foot and lift it with control, keeping your
inner thigh facing upwards and your knee soft.
Then, *slowly* lower your right leg. Repeat for the
recommended reps, then change legs.

Push your heel
away from the
floor as you lift it

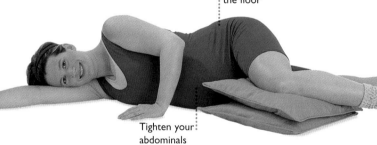

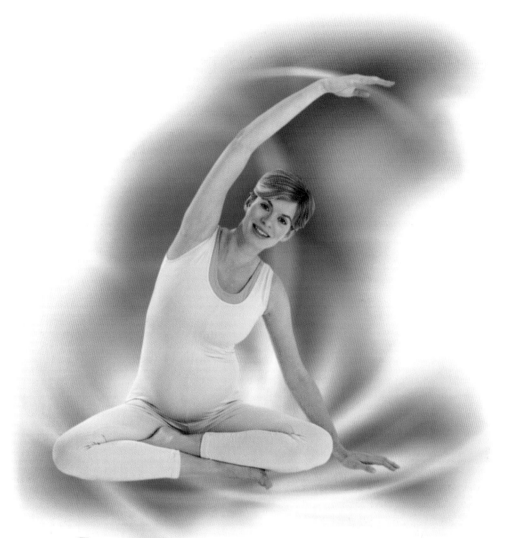

STRETCHING
AND RELAXING

It is important to give your body a chance to recover fully after your workout, so I have devoted the final part of this exercise programme to stretching and relaxation techniques. The stretches should be appropriate to the type of exercise you have just completed, so that all the muscles you have worked are returned to their original length. The relaxation exercises should follow the stretches in a full workout, but they can also be done on their own, so use every opportunity to switch off, whether it is at the end of your workout, on the train or during a break at the office.

Seated hamstring stretch

To stretch and lengthen the muscles at the back of your thighs

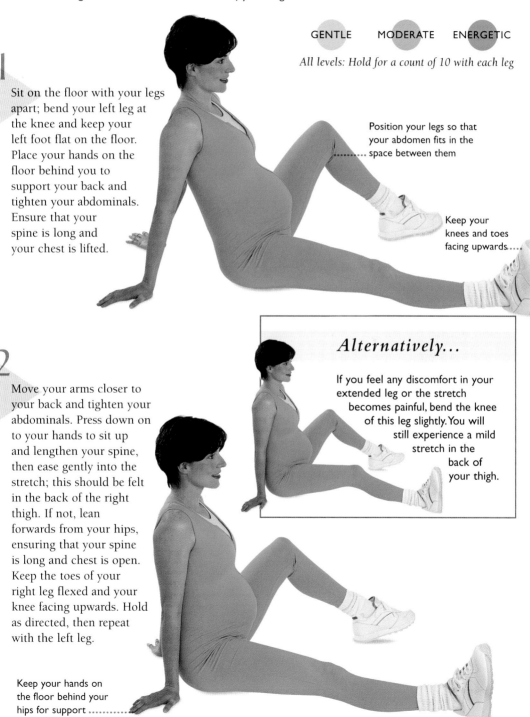

GENTLE   MODERATE   ENERGETIC

All levels: Hold for a count of 10 with each leg

1

Sit on the floor with your legs apart; bend your left leg at the knee and keep your left foot flat on the floor. Place your hands on the floor behind you to support your back and tighten your abdominals. Ensure that your spine is long and your chest is lifted.

Position your legs so that your abdomen fits in the space between them

Keep your knees and toes facing upwards

2

Move your arms closer to your back and tighten your abdominals. Press down on to your hands to sit up and lengthen your spine, then ease gently into the stretch; this should be felt in the back of the right thigh. If not, lean forwards from your hips, ensuring that your spine is long and chest is open. Keep the toes of your right leg flexed and your knee facing upwards. Hold as directed, then repeat with the left leg.

Keep your hands on the floor behind your hips for support

Alternatively...

If you feel any discomfort in your extended leg or the stretch becomes painful, bend the knee of this leg slightly. You will still experience a mild stretch in the back of your thigh.

FIRST TRIMESTER ONLY

Lying hamstring stretch

To stretch and lengthen the muscles at the back of your thighs

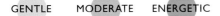

GENTLE   MODERATE   ENERGETIC

All levels: Hold for a count of 10 with each leg

1

Lie down on your back with your knees bent and your feet flat on the floor.

CAUTION

If you feel dizzy or nauseous at any stage, you *must* avoid all the exercises which involve lying on your back. Try the seated version of this exercise instead (*see page 57*).

Ensure that both buttocks are flat on the floor

Avoid pointing your toes too strongly

2

Tighten your abdominals and gently lift your left leg off the floor, keeping your knee bent. Then, take hold of the back of your thigh with both hands.

If your leg begins to tremble lower it and begin the stretch again more slowly

3

Slowly begin to straighten your left leg until you feel a stretch in the back of your left thigh. Slide one hand down to your left calf muscle to support the lower leg, if necessary. Hold as instructed, then gently lower your leg to the floor. Repeat with the right leg.

Ease slowly into the stretch; do not bounce your leg

Relax your upper body

Seated adductor stretch

To stretch and lengthen your inner thigh muscles

GENTLE   MODERATE   ENERGETIC

Hold for a count of 10; repeat if desired

1

Sit on the floor with your knees bent and the soles of your feet together. Place your hands on the floor behind you for support. Keeping your pelvis tilted and abdominal muscles tight, lengthen your spine, and sit tall.

Don't lock ....
out your elbows

2

Keeping your weight slightly forwards, move your hands closer to your body and gently slide your buttocks towards your heels until you feel a stretch in your inner thighs. Keep your spine long, your shoulders down and your abdominals tight. Hold as directed.

... Remember to keep breathing throughout

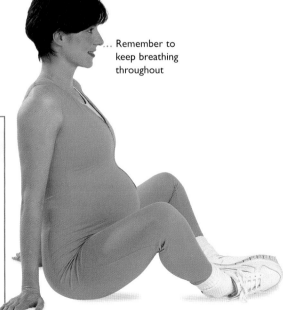

Alternatively...

If this exercise feels uncomfortable sitting with your arms behind you, rest your hands on your heels, ensuring that you keep your spine long. You may find it more comfortable if you relax your upper body forwards.

Seated gluteal stretch

To stretch and lengthen your buttock and outer thigh muscles

GENTLE   MODERATE   ENERGETIC

All levels: Hold for a count of 10 on each side

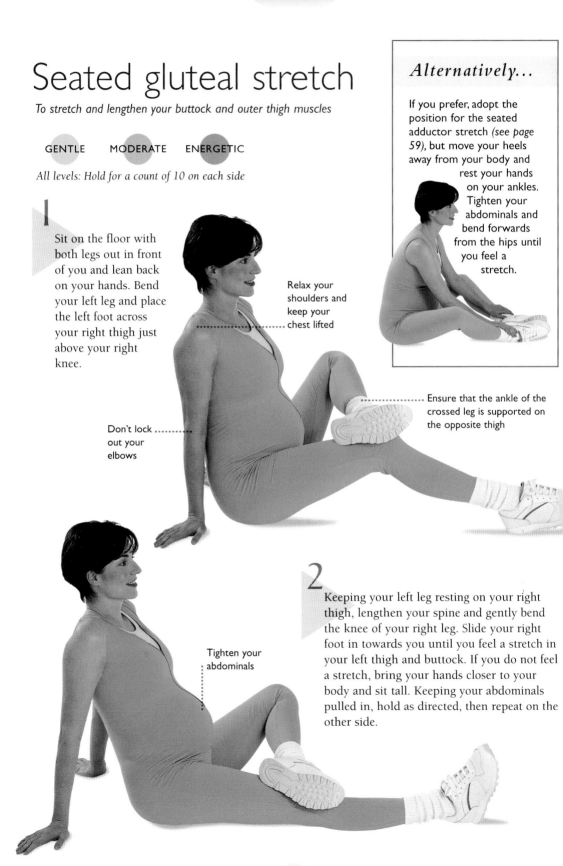

1 Sit on the floor with both legs out in front of you and lean back on your hands. Bend your left leg and place the left foot across your right thigh just above your right knee.

Relax your shoulders and keep your chest lifted

Don't lock out your elbows

Ensure that the ankle of the crossed leg is supported on the opposite thigh

Tighten your abdominals

2 Keeping your left leg resting on your right thigh, lengthen your spine and gently bend the knee of your right leg. Slide your right foot in towards you until you feel a stretch in your left thigh and buttock. If you do not feel a stretch, bring your hands closer to your body and sit tall. Keeping your abdominals pulled in, hold as directed, then repeat on the other side.

Alternatively...

If you prefer, adopt the position for the seated adductor stretch (*see page 59*), but move your heels away from your body and rest your hands on your ankles. Tighten your abdominals and bend forwards from the hips until you feel a stretch.

Seated pectoral stretch

To stretch and lengthen your chest muscles, which will improve your posture

GENTLE   MODERATE   ENERGETIC

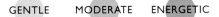

Hold for a count of 6; repeat if desired

1

Sit on the floor in a comfortable position. Rest your hands on your buttocks, tighten your abdominal muscles to lift your baby and sit tall.

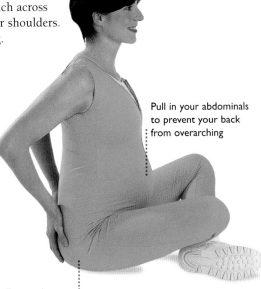

Lengthen your neck and keep it in line with your spine

Sit tall with your hands on your buttocks ....

2

Lengthen your spine, lift your chest and slowly draw your elbows back, squeezing your shoulder blades together. Hold as directed. You should feel a stretch across your chest and the front of your shoulders. Ensure that you keep breathing.

Pull in your abdominals to prevent your back from overarching

Alternatively...

You may prefer to do this stretch standing (see page 19). If so, stand with your feet hip-width apart and rest your hands on your buttocks. Slowly draw your elbows back (as described above), keeping your pelvis tilted and abdominals tight to protect your back.

Ensure that your buttocks remain flat on the floor

61

Seated triceps stretch

To stretch and lengthen the muscles at the back of your upper arms

GENTLE   MODERATE   ENERGETIC

Hold for a count of 8 with each arm

1

Sit in a comfortable position. Tighten your abdominal muscles and sit tall. Lift your right arm up to the ceiling and bend the elbow so your fingers are between your shoulder blades and pointing downwards.

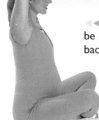

Don't forget...

◀◀◀ During this exercise you must be careful not to overarch your back. To do this, ensure that your abdominal muscles remain tight and your pelvis is tilted throughout this exercise; keep your head lifted, the spine long and in line with your neck and sit tall.

If your back does begin to overarch when performing this exercise, or if the stretch feels uncomfortable, try supporting your upper arm with your opposite hand from the front. Or, if you prefer, you can perform this stretch standing with your feet hip-width apart (see page 16). ▶▶▶

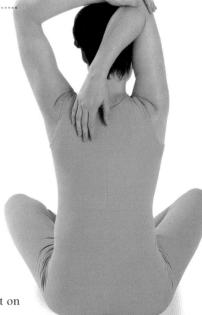

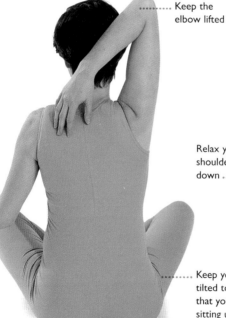

Keep the elbow lifted

Relax your shoulders down ....

Keep your pelvis tilted to ensure that you remain sitting upright

2

Take hold of your arm with your left hand and ease the elbow gently behind your head. Re-tilt your pelvis and feel the stretch in the back of your right upper arm. Hold as recommended, then repeat on the other side.

Seated side stretch

To stretch and lengthen the latissimus dorsi and obliques

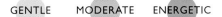

GENTLE   MODERATE   ENERGETIC

All levels: Hold for a count of 6 on each side, repeat if desired

1 Sit in a comfortable position. Tilt your pelvis and sit tall. Reach your right arm up to the ceiling and lengthen your spine. Place your left hand on the floor for extra support.

Reach your arm up to the ceiling

Soften your elbow and relax your arm

Don't forget...

Position your arm slightly in front of your body to avoid overarching your back. Be careful not to bend over too far if you feel any discomfort in your abdomen. If you prefer, you can do this exercise in a standing position (see page 15).

2 Slowly bend over to your left side, keeping your buttocks in contact with the floor and reach your right arm up and over your head. Pull in your abdominals and tilt your pelvis. Hold as instructed, then repeat on the other side.

Keep the arm long

Feel the stretch down your side

Press your shoulders down firmly

Tighten your abdominals

Take your arm further to one side as you bend

Relaxation

sitting on the floor using cushions

GENTLE   MODERATE   ENERGETIC

Allow 5–20 minutes (including waking up)

Relaxation after the more vigorous sections of this workout can lessen fatigue, release muscular tension and calm your mind. It may also help you to control pain during labour. During these exercises, ensure that all your joints are well supported and you are in a comfortable position.

Lean on two cushions to support your back

Ensure that your knees remain slightly bent

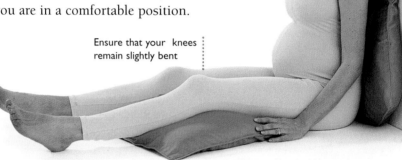

1 Sit on the floor with your back against a wall and your legs out in front of you. Place one cushion under your knees, one behind your head and another behind your lower back for support. Adjust your position until you feel really comfortable and well supported by the cushions.

Press your hea gently down into the cushio then release

2 Move your shoulders down and away from your ears and take your elbows away from your sides, then let go. Open your hands and stretch your fingers then let go. Flex your feet, then release. Separate your teeth and release the jaw. Release any tension in your forehead and close your eyes. Breathe gently and feel yourself slowly sinking into the support. Focus you thoughts on something that makes you feel calm. Remain like this for as long as possible then follow the waking up exercise (*see page 66*).

Allow your feet and ankles to roll outwards............

Roll your legs outwards from the hips

other relaxation positions

sitting in a chair

1

Sit in a comfortable chair and rest your feet on a large cushion. Place one cushion behind your lower back and another behind your head for support. Rest your arms on the sides of the chair and lie your head back on the cushion.

2

Move your shoulders down, away from your ears and lift your elbows away from the chair, then let go. Open your hands and stretch your fingers, then let go. Let your legs roll outward from the hips. Flex your feet, then let go. Separate your teeth and release the jaw. Release any tension in your forehead and close your eyes. Breathe gently and feel yourself sinking into the support as you exhale. Think about something calming.

lying with one knee bent

1

Lie on your side on the floor with your top leg bent and the other leg straight. Place a large cushion or cushions underneath your top knee and thigh to reduce discomfort in your lower back. Bend your arms and place them on the floor in front of you. Place a cushion under your head (and under your abdomen, if required).

2

Move your top shoulder down and away from your ear and lift your elbow off the floor, then let go. Open your hands and stretch your fingers, then let go. Flex your feet, then release. Separate your teeth and release the jaw. Release any tension in your forehead and close your eyes. Breathe gently and feel yourself sinking into the support with each breath out. Focus your thoughts on something that makes you feel calm.

lying with both knees bent

1

Lie on your side on the floor with both knees bent up, one on top of the other, and your back gently curved. Bend your arms and place them in front of you for support. Place one cushion under your head and another between your knees. Relax your abdomen and ensure that your body weight is slightly forwards.

2

Move your top shoulder down, away from your ear and lift your elbow off the floor, then let go. Open your hands and stretch your fingers, then let go. Flex your feet, then release. Separate your teeth and release the jaw. Release any tension in your forehead and close your eyes. Breathe gently and feel yourself sinking into the support with each breath out. Think about something calming. Remain in this position for as long as possible.

waking up

1
Remain in your chosen relaxation position
(*see pages 64-65*) and perform your pelvic
floor exercises: one slow contraction,
followed by four quick ones (*see page 43*).
Gently rotate your wrists and ankles in slow
circular movements. Take care *not* to point
your toes as this may cause cramp in your
feet and calf muscles. Now, stretch and bend
your fingers.

Relax your
abdominal
muscles

2
Stretch your top arm up above your head,
then relax. Stretch your top leg away from
your body, without pointing your toes, then
relax. Stretch out your arm and leg together,
then release. (If you are seated, repeat the
stretches on both sides.)

Relax the
lower leg

3
When you feel ready to get up, place both
hands flat on the floor in front of you and
gently push yourself up into a side kneeling
position. Slowly move up to a seated
position, keeping your knees and feet
together. Remain in this position to perform
the remobilizing exercises (*see pages
67–68*) before slowly standing up (*see
page 69*).

Keep your shoulders
down and relaxed

CAUTION

You must allow yourself
enough time to recover and
find your bearings after
relaxing. Standing up
suddenly may cause you
to feel dizzy and light-
headed.

Ensure that
your feet are
together

Remobilizing

ankle mobility

GENTLE   **MODERATE**   **ENERGETIC**

Allow 5–10 minutes (including standing up)

After your relaxation session it is important to allow your body sufficient time to wake-up before standing up. This waking up period reduces the risk of experiencing dizziness and leaves you feeling more alert and refreshed.

Lengthen
your neck
.... and spine

Ensure that
your knees
remain soft

Tighten your
abdominals ....

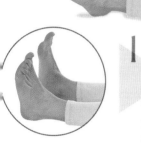

1 Sit with your legs out in front of you and lean back on your hands. Flex your feet so that your toes move towards the ceiling and your heels push away from you; release and repeat 3 or 4 times.

2 Gently rotate your ankles in large circular movements; don't point your toes as this may cause cramp in your feet and calf muscles. Repeat slowly 3 or 4 times, then change the direction of the circle.

Open your
chest and relax
your shoulders ....

Keep your ....
toes relaxed

other remobilizing exercises

shoulder rolls

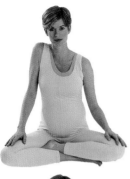

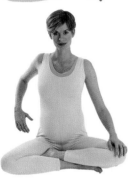

1

Sit tall in a comfortable position. Tilt your pelvis and tighten your abdominals to lift your baby. Relax your hands on your knees and press your shoulders down gently. Rotate your right shoulder forwards, then raise it towards your ear.

2

Circle the shoulder behind you in a large, exaggerated manner, taking it back and down again. Keep your abdominals pulled in and the rest of your body still. Do 8 reps with your right shoulder, then repeat on the other side.

neck mobility

1

Sit in a comfortable position with your pelvis tilted and abdominals tight. Rest your hands on your knees, press your shoulders down and lengthen your spine.

2

Slowly tilt your head over to the left side, pressing your ear towards your shoulder. Do *not* be tempted to raise your shoulder towards your ear. Pause, then return to the upright position before repeating on the right side.

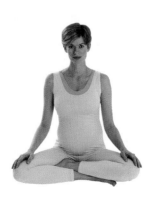

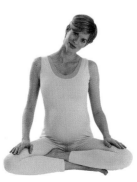

side reach

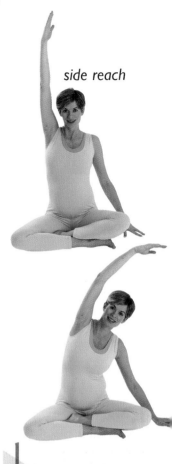

1

Sit in a comfortable position. Tilt your pelvis, tighten your abdominal muscles to lift your baby and sit tall. Place your left hand on the floor beside you for support and reach your right arm up towards the ceiling, keeping your spine long.

2

Slowly bend over to the left side, keeping your arm slightly forwards to prevent your back from arching. Feel a stretch down your right side. Hold for 6 counts, then lower your arm and sit tall before repeating with your left arm.

standing up

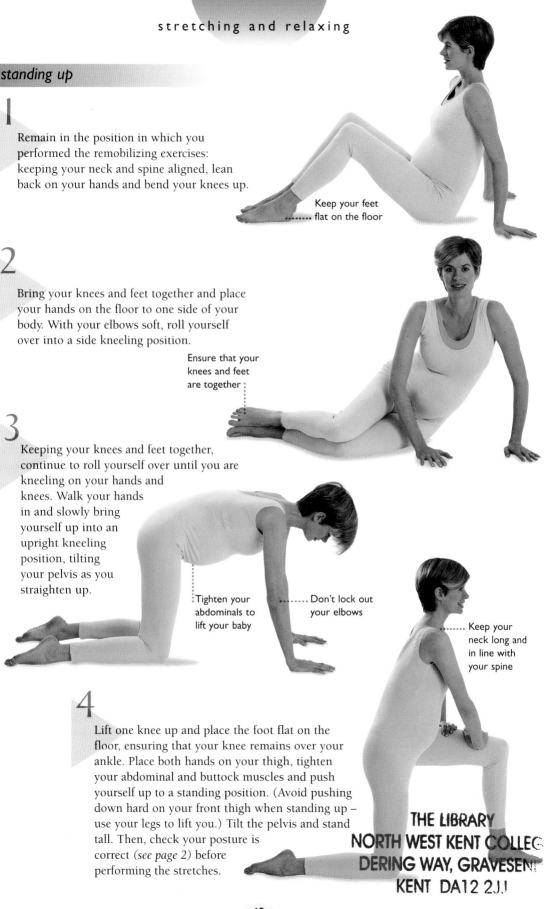

1

Remain in the position in which you performed the remobilizing exercises: keeping your neck and spine aligned, lean back on your hands and bend your knees up.

Keep your feet
········ flat on the floor

2

Bring your knees and feet together and place your hands on the floor to one side of your body. With your elbows soft, roll yourself over into a side kneeling position.

Ensure that your
knees and feet
are together :

3

Keeping your knees and feet together, continue to roll yourself over until you are kneeling on your hands and knees. Walk your hands in and slowly bring yourself up into an upright kneeling position, tilting your pelvis as you straighten up.

Tighten your
abdominals to
lift your baby

········ Don't lock out
your elbows

········ Keep your
neck long and
in line with
your spine

4

Lift one knee up and place the foot flat on the floor, ensuring that your knee remains over your ankle. Place both hands on your thigh, tighten your abdominal and buttock muscles and push yourself up to a standing position. (Avoid pushing down hard on your front thigh when standing up – use your legs to lift you.) Tilt the pelvis and stand tall. Then, check your posture is correct (*see page 2*) before performing the stretches.

Calf stretch

To stretch and lengthen the calf muscle. This can be particularly helpful if you suffer from cramp

GENTLE   MODERATE   ENERGETIC

Hold for a count of 8 on each side

Tighten your................
abdominals

Rest your hand on
the back of a sturdy
.... chair for support

1 Stand with your left side to a chair and place your left hand on the back of it for support.

Ensure that
your feet are
flat on the floor ....

2 With your feet about hip-width apart and facing forwards, take a step backwards with your right foot; keep your left knee soft and lengthen your spine.

3 Bend your left leg and straighten your right leg, gently pressing the right heel into the floor. Keep your weight forward to maintain a diagonal line from your head to your heel. Re-tilt your pelvis and lift your baby up and in towards you. If you cannot feel the stretch, move your right foot further back. Hold as directed, then change legs.

Keep your........
pelvis tilted

Feel the
stretch in the
bulky part of
your calf

70

Quadriceps stretch

To stretch and lengthen the muscles at the front of your thighs

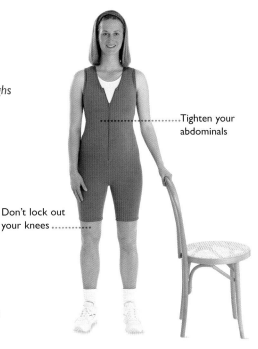

Tighten your abdominals

GENTLE   MODERATE   ENERGETIC

Hold for a count of 8 on each side

Don't lock out your knees

1

Stand sideways to a chair and rest one hand on the back of it for support. With your feet about hip-width apart, transfer your weight on to your left leg, lifting through the supporting hip. Tilt your pelvis and stand tall.

2

With your left leg bent, lift your right knee up in front of you. Then, hold your right ankle with your right hand at the front.

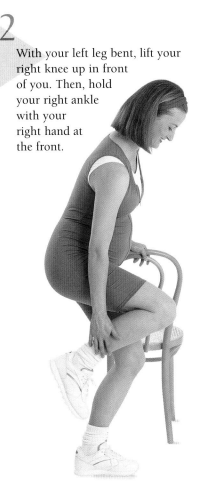

3

Move your right knee back until it aligns with the hip and lift up through your left leg. Tilt your pelvis, tighten your abdominals and lengthen your spine. If you do not feel a stretch in the front of your right thigh, move the leg gently behind you and re-tilt your pelvis. Hold as directed, then change legs.

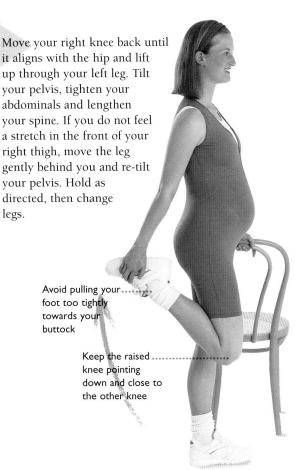

Avoid pulling your foot too tightly towards your buttock

Keep the raised knee pointing down and close to the other knee

Hip stretch

To stretch and lengthen the hip flexors (muscles at the front of your hips), which often tighten during pregnancy. Regularly stretching these muscles will help you to maintain a good pelvic tilt

GENTLE   MODERATE   ENERGETIC

Hold for a count of 6 on each side

Tighten your abdominals

1

Stand with your left side to a sturdy chair and rest your hand on the back of it for support. Tilt your pelvis and stand tall.

2

With your feet hip-width apart, step your right leg back with both feet facing forwards and lift your right heel off the floor. Keep your back long, tighten your abdominals to lift your baby and make sure that your weight is central between both feet.

Lift up from the hips to keep them correctly aligned

3

Bend both knees and do an exaggerated pelvic tilt, lifting your hips up at the front and bringing your bottom under you. Lengthen your spine and open your chest. Pull in your abdominals to secure the stretch, which should be felt at the front of the hip of your right leg. If you do not feel a stretch, re-tilt your pelvis and lengthen your spine further. Hold as directed, then repeat with the left leg.

Keep your body weight balanced between both feet

Upward reach

To stretch the latissimus dorsi (muscles down your sides) and to finish your exercise session with a long spine and perfect posture

GENTLE   MODERATE   ENERGETIC

Hold for a count of 3 on each side

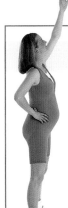

Don't forget...

To prevent your back from arching, ensure that your raised arm is slightly in front of your body and your weight is forwards; this is especially important during your third trimester. Leaning back during this exercise may place unnecessary stress on your lower back, leading to back pain.

1

Stand with your feet slightly wider than the hips and rest your left hand on your hip. Tighten your abdominals to lift your baby and stand tall.

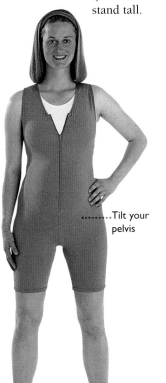

............Tilt your pelvis

Keep your feet wide to provide .....a stable base

2

Reach up to the ceiling with your right arm, lengthen your spine and extend the arm up as high as you can. Keep your body weight slightly forwards and tighten your abdominals. Lower your arm, relax your shoulders down and stand tall. Repeat with your left arm.

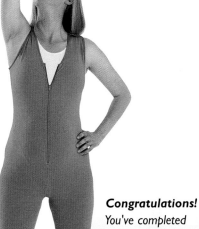

Ensure that your knees are soft ....

Balance your weight between both feet ....

Congratulations!
You've completed your workout for today. I hope you are feeling refreshed and invigorated. It's now time to drink a glass of water and to enjoy a healthy snack to replenish your energy levels.

INDEX

ACKNOWLEDGEMENTS

CARROLL & BROWN would very much like to thank: Professor Jim Clapp for reviewing the manuscript; Storm, Pregnant Pause and Bubblegum modelling agencies; and Fit for 2 for providing the clothing.

PICTURE CREDITS p.viii & p.xvii Pictor International Ltd